The Entsminger Guide to Prehospital 12-Lead Electrocardiogram Interpretation

Nick Entsminger

The Entsminger Guide to Prehospital 12-Lead Electrocardiogram Interpretation

Nick Entsminger, Author and illustrator

Graham Hewson, Editor

Copyright © 2020 by Nicholas Neal Entsminger. All rights reserved.

P.O. Box 132
Bridgeville, CA 95526

All rights reserved. This book is protected by copyright. No part of this book may be reproduced in any form, including photocopying, recording, or other electronic or mechanical methods, without written permission from the copyright owner, except in the case of brief quotations embodied in reviews and certain other non-commercial uses permitted by copyright law.

Library of Congress Control Number: 2020906079

ISBN: 978-0-578-67174-1

DISCLAIMER

The author and editor have made an honest effort to ensure the originality of this textbook. The diagnostic and treatment modalities contained within this text follow current recommendations and practice at publication. However, given ongoing research, changes in government and regional medical authority protocols—and the constant flow of information relating to ECG interpretation and treatment within the prehospital setting—the reader is urged to refer to their regional protocols and diagnostic requirements to ensure compliance.

An effort was taken to confirm the accuracy of this text and describe generally accepted interpretative and treatment practices. Neither the author nor the editor is responsible for errors, omissions, or any consequences from applying the information in this text, making no warranty, expressed or implied, concerning the currency, completeness, or accuracy of the contents of this publication. Application of this information remains the professional responsibility of the practitioner, as the clinical treatments included may not be considered absolute and universal recommendations.

For Brooke, Annabelle, and Dad

Brooke: *Thank you for your patience and encouragement during the unremitting onslaught of self-critique, doubt, and deprecation. As with most things, you deserve far more credit than you receive. You are my rock—keeping my focus midst the torrent of disparagement.*

Annabelle: *If this book has any worth, I hope that it shows you the importance of risk. Without risk, one cannot fail; and without failure, one cannot better themselves. Know that those who sit quietly amid loud voices cannot silence ignorance. Never fear that which a skeptic wouldn't attempt, and take comfort that Dad will cheer you all the way—no matter the outcome.*

Dad: *For all the dreams you never grasped, and all that I wish to tell you. I hope this text offers a small sense of pride as you experience wonders only imagined by those who miss you.*

$$\text{Ego} = \frac{1}{\text{knowledge}} :$$

*The more the knowledge,
lesser the ego.*

*Lesser the knowledge,
more the ego."*

- Albert Einstein

Acknowledgments

I would like to thank those whom I have worked with over the years for their continuous instruction and support of my pursuits. Without them, this text would not have come to fruition. Additionally, I would like to credit Graham Hewson in ushering clarity to this text through his skill in the English language. Finally, this book wouldn't have been completed without the love and support of my wife and her long years of encouragement, enhanced affectionately by the smiling face and laughter of my beautiful daughter.

Table of Contents

Preface

Chapter 1: Lead Types and Placement in the Prehospital Setting.................. 1

Chapter 2: Evolution of a Myocardial Infarction........................ 6

Chapter 3: Print layout, Lead Associations, and Acute Coronary Diagnostic Criteria for Field Personnel.................... 11

Chapter 4: Cardiac Axis and Blocks For EMS........................ 27

Chapter 5: Field Interpretation: *The Meat and Potatoes* of What You Need to Know...................... 36

Chapter 6: The LEADS Approach to Prehospital 12-Lead EKG Interpretation................................ 56

Chapter 7: Calling the Hospital with a Cardiac Patient: The Dos and *Don'ts*.................................. 125

Acronym Glossary... 133

References.. 135

Preface

In recent years, the 12-lead electrocardiogram (EKG) has become an integral part of prehospital emergency care. The EKG's addition to the scope of practice of advanced life support providers has given prehospital personnel a long needed and overdue tool to diagnose acute cardiac events by expanding the assessable surface area of the heart by adding an additional 8 vantage points to the tradition 3-lead EKG. This critical addition has aided significantly in survival rates across the nation. Although some systems still require EKG transmission to a respective base hospital before or during transport, it's essential that prehospital providers have a solid understanding of 12-lead EKG interpretation for the benefit of their patients and the EMS profession as a whole.

This guide was developed to instruct prehospital providers to recognize a cardiac event in the adult population utilizing the 12-lead EKG, and to understand the basic underlying principles that allow for the EKG's function. The text assumes readers have a fundamental understanding of QRS morphology, 3-lead interpretation, and the physiology of the heart. After completion of this short treatise, readers will have an understanding of the 12-lead EKG, and this knowledge will promote the general importance of the emergency medical services profession throughout the medical community.

Furthermore, I wish to help prehospital professionals to learn and flourish in their practice, not only in the realm of cardiac care, but in every aspect of the profession. Experience dictates that progress is built on the foundations of trust and confidence in less than ideal situations when knowledge, critical thinking skills, and actions reign true. This describes, perfectly, the EMS and prehospital environment.

1

Lead Types and Placement in the Prehospital Setting

Before the addition of the 12-lead EKG, paramedics were reliant on the 3-lead version. The 3-lead was simple, easy to place, and effective at identifying arrhythmias, though, despite its ease, was ineffective at revealing infarctions to a large portion of the heart. As prehospital medicine advanced, the 12-lead EKG solved many of the problems associated with 3-lead reads. Although the 12-lead is widely used today, many advanced life support personnel still don't understand the basics required for its use, either because the skill remains outside their comfort zone or they haven't had the opportunity to learn it. This chapter presents a simple approach to EKG functions.

Introduction

The 12-lead EKG uses two vantages to gather information: one that looks from the atrioventricular (AV) node toward the apex of the heart; and the other that looks from the AV node toward the left ventricle as it depolarizes. Electrodes placed at these two vantage points gather the most information because the normal electrical pathway travels from the AV node down toward the left hip through the apex of the heart, and outward toward the left breast, giving preference to the left ventricle (*figure 1.1*). These two pathways are separated on the EKG printout (*figure 1.2, next page*): the tracings to the left of the printout's midline look down toward the left hip, and these are the *frontal leads*; tracings shown on the right side of the EKG looks outward toward the left breast, and these lead tracings are termed the *horizontal* or *precordial leads*.

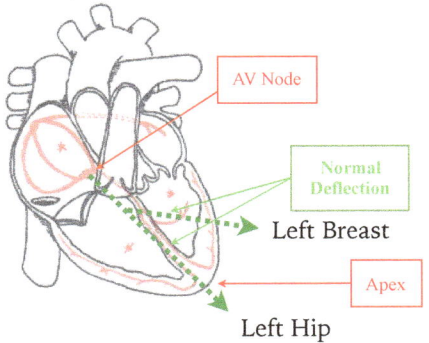

Figure 1.1: *Depolarization Pathways of the Heart Favoring the Left Ventricle.*

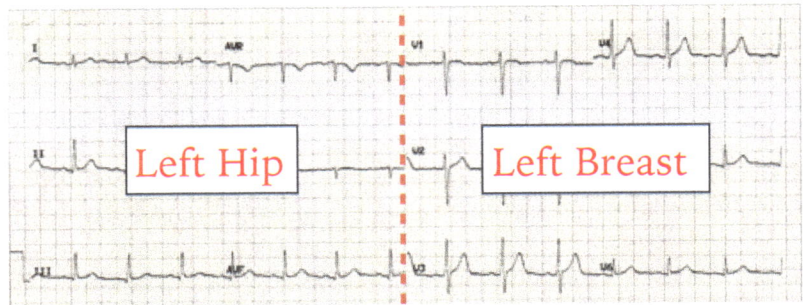

Figure 1.2: *Printout identifying the separation of vantages on the 12-Lead EKG (Adapted from Normal 12-Lead EKG, in Life in the Fast Lane, Retrieved February 8, 2017, from litfl.com, Copyright 2017 by Mike Cadogan. Reprinted with permission).*

Precordial leads are referred to as horizontal within this text, as this gives a better understanding of the impulse direction they read.

Electrode Versus Lead

An electrode and a lead are not the same. An electrode adhered to the body surface is responsible for receiving an electrical impulse originating from the AV node, while a lead is the path between a given electrode and the AV impulse. For example, lead II requires an electrode placed on the right shoulder and the left hip area. The lead is an imaginative line of sight between these two electrodes respective to the trajectory of the AV impulse within the heart muscle. The electrodes receive the information, while the lead is the route between the two electrodes. Think of the electrodes as the start and finish markers on a map and the lead is the trail needed to get from one to the next. Some leads vary in the number of electrodes they use depending on the surface area they are viewing: some utilize one electrode, others two.

Frontal Leads

The frontal leads are the standard 3-lead EKG of the past, measuring conduction from the AV node down to the apex of the heart. Place the palm of your hand over your heart and slide it diagonally down to your left hip; this is the plane read by these leads. Leads I, II, and III use two electrodes—one positive and one negative—to receive information (*figure 1.3*). Because of this, they are referred to as *bipolar leads* (*bi* meaning two). The positive electrode of a given lead is the primary receiver. Lead I looks from the

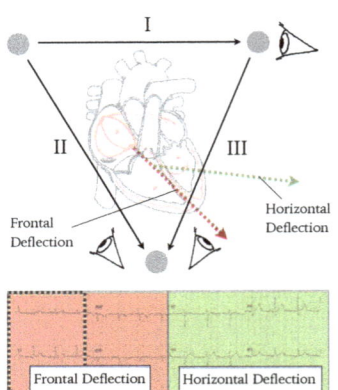

Figure 1.3: *Vantage Points of Frontal Leads I-III in Relation to the Normal AV Deflection and Their Representative Space on the 12-Lead EKG Printout. (EKG from Normal 12-Lead EKG, in Life in the Fast Lane, Retrieved February 8, 2017 from litfl.com. Copyright 2017 by Mike Cadogan. Reprinted with permission).*

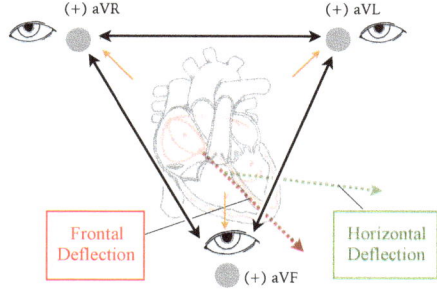

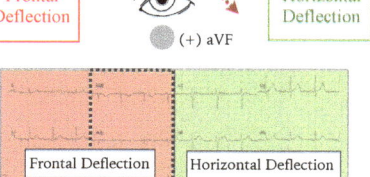

Figure 1.4: *Vantage Points of the Augmented Frontal Leads in Relation to the Normal Deflection of the AV Node Including Their Corresponding Representative Space on the EKG Printout.*

negative electrode on the right shoulder toward the positive electrode on the left shoulder; lead II looks from the negative right shoulder to toward the positive left hip; lead III looks from the negative left shoulder to the positive left hip. Each lead gives a specific vantage to measure the conduction leaving the AV node.

The frontal leads also include a second set of leads, termed the *augmented* frontal leads. These leads include aVR, aVL, and aVF. These leads use the same frontal plane as leads I, II, and III, yet use one positive electrode (*uni* means one) measuring the deflection between the remaining two negative electrodes (*figure 1.4*). These leads aid further in identifying the direction of the impulse and any alterations to it. They also offer information on additional regions of the heart not seen using the standard 3-lead EKG (discussed in Chapter 3).

Horizontal Leads

The horizontal leads, V_1 - V_6, are located on the right side of the EKG printout. They're termed *horizontal* because their vantage point is roughly horizontal to the AV node (*figure 1.5*). Place your right palm over your sternum and slide it around your left side under your left armpit. This movement represents the perspective of the horizontal leads.

V_1-V_6 use one positive electrode and termed *unipolar* like the augmented leads, yet the horizontal leads have no negative reference. Standard placement of the horizontal leads focuses on the left ventricle, since this is the most important chamber for systemic profusion.

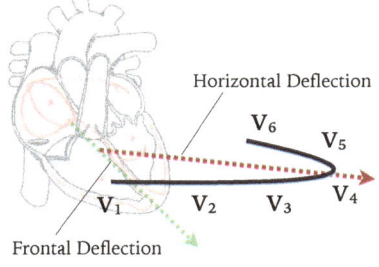

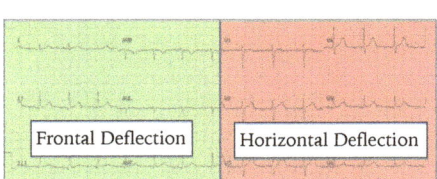

Figure 1.5: *Vantage Points of the Horizontal Leads in Relation to Normal Deflection Dispersement of the AV Node Including Their Corresponding Representative Space on the EKG Printout.*

Affixing the Electrodes

Prehospital medical personnel know the phrase *"white on right, smoke over fire"* for placement of the frontal leads. Assuming this general knowledge, we'll focus on the placement of the horizontal leads realizing that textbook placement of these electrodes is often not feasible in the chaotic realm of prehospital emergency medical care. The following is the most expedient placement technique for prehospital providers to achieve a relatively precise reading.

The easiest way to place the horizontal leads is first to find the sternum (*figure 1.6*). Place V_1 on the right side of the sternum and V_2 on the left, both just off the bone and about a one-third the way up from the xiphoid process. From here, place lead V_4 just under the left nipple (adjust for girth and breast size). Next, place lead V_6 on the axilla at the level of V_1 and V_2. Finally, fill in the remaining leads, V_3 and V_5, equidistant to their neighbor electrodes. This technique is a down-and-dirty way to place your electrodes quickly and give you an accurate representation of the electrophysiology of the heart in the prehospital setting.

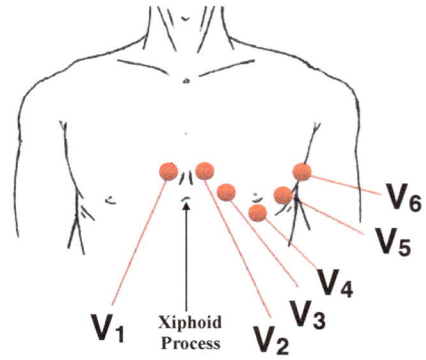

Figure 1.6: *Proper Electrode Placement of the Precordial Leads.*

A fundamental understanding of the lead types and placement of the 12-lead EKG is essential for understanding the morphologies displayed on it. It's the electrode placement of the positive electrodes, in relation to the impulse as it travels through the tissue, that gives you the readout you see on the monitor and printout. Any muscle damage between the AV node and positive electrode of a given lead will alter the impulse pattern read by the positive leads on the 12-lead EKG, as will inaccurate electrode placement.

Takeaway Notes from Chapter 1:

- *The 12-lead EKG is comprised of two types of leads over two different planes: the frontal leads, bipolar I, II, III, and augmented, unipolar aVR, aVL, and aVF, and the horizontal leads, precordial leads V_1 - V_6. The easiest way to memorize these planes is to understand that the frontal leads measure impulses from top to bottom and the horizontal leads measure from the back to the front.*

2

Evolution of a Myocardial Infarction

Recognizing an acute myocardial event is crucial to prehospital cardiac care, yet equally critical is the recognition that a cardiac patient will more commonly present with a normal 12-lead EKG. Less than fifty percent of patients with symptoms of an acute coronary event will have findings on their first EKG, and, of these patients, ten percent will prove to have had an acute myocardial infarction (MI) through diagnostic laboratory testing or interventional imaging with any subsequent EKG change. In fact, most cardiac patients will never present with any abnormal findings on their EKG. Prehospital providers must *never* forget the adage, *Treat the patient, not the monitor.* If you have a high level of suspicion, act on it! Additionally, ALS personnel should never trust their monitor's interpretation; it is often wrong or vague in its findings, lending to a need for a strong skillset in reading and understanding the 12-lead EKG. Knowledge of physical symptoms and exam findings will aid prehospital providers in effectively identifying a cardiac occurrence early in its progression.

Quick Terminology Review

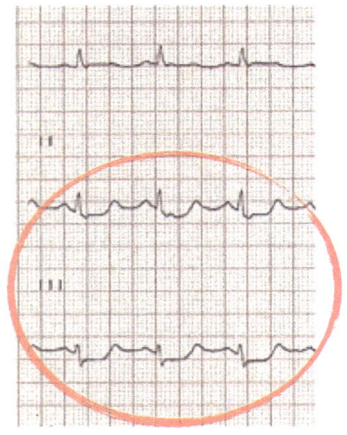

Figure 2.1: *Inferior NSTEMI Represented by ST Depression in the Frontal Leads II and III.*

There are two types of acute coronary events: non-ST elevation myocardial infarction (NSTEMI) and ST elevation myocardial infarction (STEMI). NSTEMI patients represent the vast majority of symptomatic cardiac patients, yet their EKG reveals either no significant findings, or findings other than ST elevation (*figure 2.1*).

NSTEMIs result from a partial occlusion of a large coronary artery, or the complete occlusion of a lesser branch of a major vessel, leading to partial thickness damage of the myocardium. Diagnosis of a NSTEMI requires laboratory testing of cardiac biomarkers such as troponin. Positive values of troponin confirm a NSTEMI, while negative results are likely due to unstable angina caused by coronary artery stenosis (narrowing) or spasm. Patients with negative biomarkers often require hospitalization for observation and retesting to ensure they don't develop positive troponin levels or ST elevation over time. This means NSTEMIs may develop into STEMIs (*figure 2.2*).

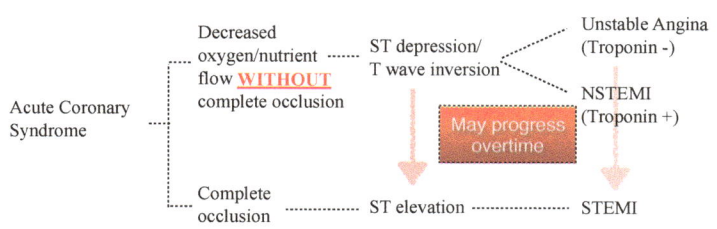

Figure 2.2: *Diagram Comparing STEMI and NSTEMI.*

In contrast, a STEMI presents on the 12-lead EKG with ST segment elevation (*figure 2.3*). A STEMI results from a complete occlusion of a large coronary artery, leading to full thickness damage of the myocardium. STEMIs require timely intervention.

An analogy to differentiate between a NSTEMI and STEMI is to think of a steady stream feeding a small pond. The water levels within the pond remain high as long as the stream continues to flow into it. Should rocks (plaque) accumulate and slow the flow of water into the pond, or completely block a smaller inlet, the pond levels will drop, partially exposing dead soil that was once underwater, but leaving some water as the flow continues at a lesser rate. This is equivalent to a NSTEMI where a partial occlusion of a major artery or a full occlusion of a smaller tributary causes partial thickness damage. Over time, rocks may continue to accumulate in the impeded area, leading to a complete obstruction of flow. Consequently, the pond will eventually dry up, as it is not being fed, exposing the murky depths that were once underwater: This is a STEMI, caused by a complete occlusion leading to full thickness damage.

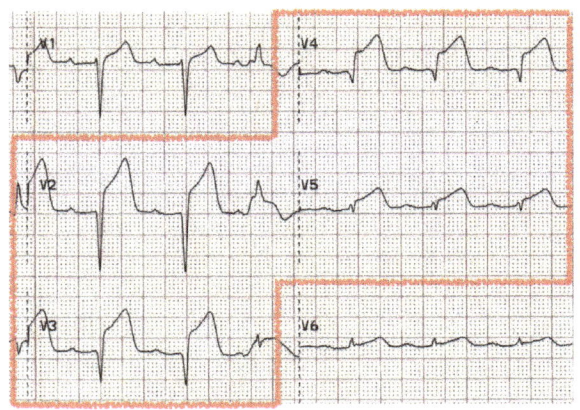

Figure 2.3: *Anterio-lateral STEMI Represented by ST Elevation with Associated First Degree Block.*

Whether a NSTEMI or STEMI, oxygen and nutrients are decreased to the myocardium, causing tissue breakdown and increasing the patient's troponin level. If not promptly remedied, obstructed cardiac muscle will suffocate and necrose. An occlusion within any coronary artery can cause damage, ranging from subtle to detrimental, depending on how much of the heart's surface area the artery supplies. For example, a complete occlusion of the left main coronary artery (LMCA) affects the entire left ventricle and is often a death sentence for an affected patient. Identification of a LMCA is discussed in Chapter 4.

QRS Morphologies During an ST Elevation Myocardial Infarction

During an MI, the morphology of the QRS complex changes with progression and time. While QRS changes are often concrete, the time length of a specific stage varies from patient to patient. Therefore, the stage you see will indicate the extent of the damage that has occurred, rather than the time that has passed. Here is a chronological breakdown of the typical stages of a STEMI:

1. The first clue is an **increased T wave height**. Upon occlusion of a coronary artery, the T wave will increase sharply in positive amplitude within minutes to hours of occlusion (*figure 2.5*). Note that this pattern may also be seen with hyperkalemic patients as well, though hyperkalemic patients will present with a diffuse pattern across the 12-lead EKG, as opposed to the regional presentation of an early STEMI.

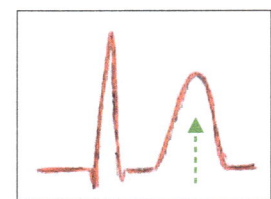

Figure 2.5: *Demonstration of a Hyperacute T Wave.*

2. As the timeframe lengthens, the **ST segment will increase in height** from the isoelectric line, representing damage to the myocardium (*figure 2.6*). During this phase, and all subsequent phases, aspirin and nitroglycerin are essential to care: aspirin for its anti-platelet congregation effects, and nitroglycerin for its vasodilatory effects.

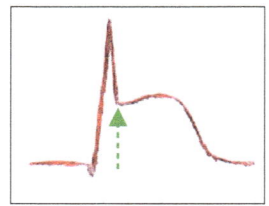

Figure 2.6: *Demonstration of ST Segment Elevation.*

3. Next, there is a **loss of clarity of the R and S waves**, as they meld and round together (*figure 2.7*). Additionally, T wave inversion and a subtle Q wave may be seen as tissue begins to die.

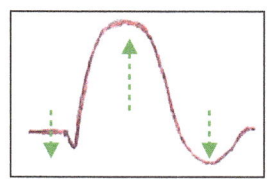

Figure 2.7: *Demonstration of Loss of R and T Wave Morphology With T Wave Inversion.*

4. If left untreated, the ST segment will return to baseline, and **a fully developed Q wave will be seen**, indicating that tissues within the region have become necrotic (*figure 2.8*). Should the patient not arrest, this Q wave will remain indefinitely and is an indicator of past infarctions on subsequent EKGs. Q wave development is a late sign, often appearing days or months after the onset of symptoms.

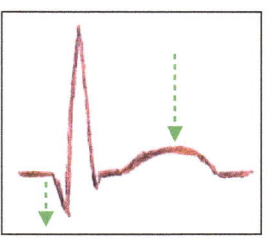

Figure 2.8: *Q Wave Formation.*

Synopsis

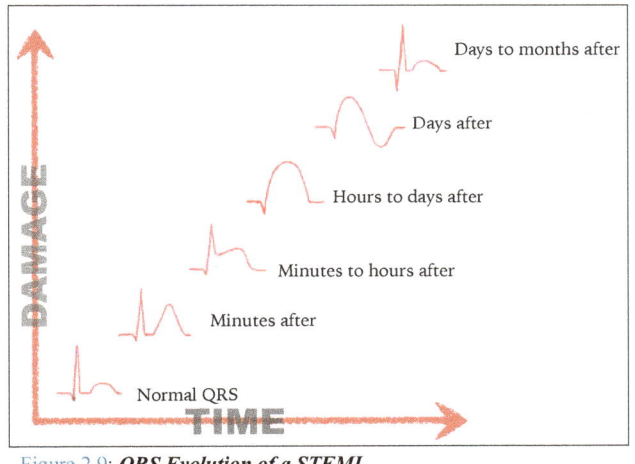

Figure 2.9: *QRS Evolution of a STEMI.*

While the manifestations of a MI are steadfast, the time frames are not (*figure 2.9*). Some patients may take hours to develop hyperacute T waves or ST elevation. Therefore, the key to an effective diagnosis is your clinical impression, history taking, and exam. Suspicion should be high in those patients with preexisting conditions that increase their risk of an acute coronary event (i.e. diabetes, hypertension, obesity, etc.), and those who look very poor on scene. A robust clinical suspicion, leading to quick intervention and transport, is better than any tool you have.

This chapter included a brief explanation of the evolution of an acute coronary event on the 12-lead EKG. Understand that acute coronary events are often difficult to identify in patients with preexisting cardiac conditions affecting normal QRS morphology (i.e., patients with implanted pacemakers, bundle branch blocks, and conditions lending to shifts in cardiac conduction angles). Bundle branch blocks are discussed further in Chapter 4. Despite these difficulties, the progressive changes explained in this chapter are essential to understand. These EKG changes assist in recognizing a myocardial infarction as well as staging and identifying the corresponding region of the infarct. The following chapter will address these concepts.

Takeaway Notes from Chapter 2:

- *A NSTEMI commonly presents with a symptomatic patient and a normal EKG or an EKG revealing ST depression or T wave inversion indicative of ischemia. These presentations are most common, so maintain a high level of suspicion when these signs are present. "Treat the patient, not the monitor!" Many of these patients require cardiac enzymes to confirm the diagnosis. Should the patient's troponin be positive, a NSTEMI is diagnosed; if negative, it is often due to unstable angina.*

- *The most common STEMI patterns on the EKG are as follows:*
  (Time ↓)
  1. *Increase in positive T wave amplitude (occlusion)*
  2. *Increase in the ST segment amplitude (injury)*
  3. *Rounded R and S waves with T wave inversion*
  4. *Decrease in ST segment elevation with T wave reversion (return to baseline)*
  5. *Formation of the Q wave (tissue death)*

- *Timeframes for QRS changes during an acute coronary event are not concrete; however, each progressive change is an indicator of the extent of tissue damage.*

3

Print Layout, Lead Associations, and Acute Coronary Diagnostic Criteria for Field Personnel

Introduction

In Chapter 2, we discussed QRS variations during the evolution of an ST elevation MI. Once the QRS patterns are understood, understanding of the 12-lead EKG layout and MI diagnostic criteria shape a means of identifying an acute coronary event in the field setting. This chapter presents these topics in a quick approach for EMS personnel.

The 12-Lead EKG Printout

There are variations of EKG print layouts depending on the monitor brand your company or agency utilizes, though the leads and interpretation remain universal. The standard layout is a rectangular page divided into 12 sections: three vertically and four horizontally, representing the 12 combinations of electrode placement. Recall from Chapter 1 that there are 10 electrodes yet 12 leads due to the amount of electrodes a given lead requires for a particular vantage: some one, others two. Similarly, remember that the electrodes are the wires, while the leads use the electrodes to give results.

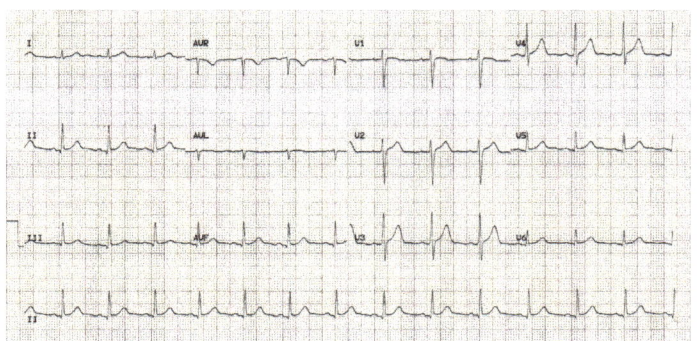

Figure 3.1: *Example of a Normal 12-Lead Electrocardiogram Printout with Lead II Shown at the Bottom of the Printout. From liftl.com.*

Each section on the printout embodies nearly a three-second read of a specified area of myocardium. Commonly, a strip of lead II and aVR is found at the bottom of the page for initial rhythm interpretation (*figure 3.1*). Cardiac axis will be discussed in a Chapter 4.

11

The Layout

As discussed in Chapter 1, the leads on the left side of the EKG are frontal leads, and those on the right are the horizontal leads. Each corresponding lead is labeled within a given section, representing an area of myocardium fed by a specific coronary artery (*figure 3.2*).

There are multiple branches of the coronary arteries, and this multiplicity can lead to confusion. Precise identification of the artery affected is not crucial for prehospital care, however a fundamental understanding is necessary because some arterial occlusions are more critical than others due to the extent of myocardium they supply. There are several methods to identify regions and arterial flow on the EKG. I'll provide a simplified approach for you in the next section.

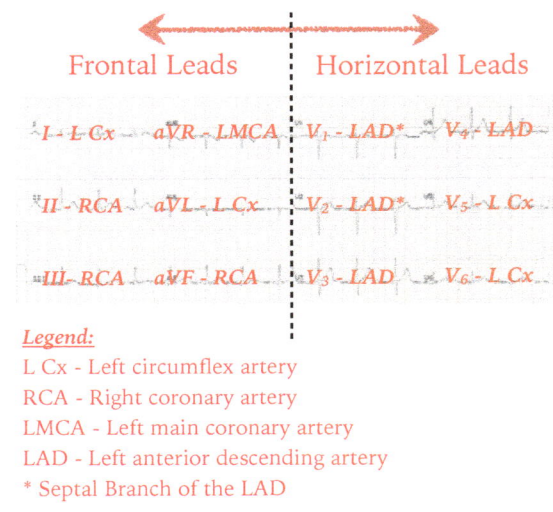

Legend:
L Cx - Left circumflex artery
RCA - Right coronary artery
LMCA - Left main coronary artery
LAD - Left anterior descending artery
* Septal Branch of the LAD

Figure 3.2: *12-Lead EKG Printout with Associated Coronary Artery Supply.*

Field Interpretation of the 12-Lead Electrocardiogram

The primary concept to understand is each lead's vantage in relation to the electrical impulse leaving the AV node. For example, leads II, III, and aVF focus on the inferior surface and right ventricle of the heart (*figure 3.3*). The right coronary artery (RCA) and its branches are the primary arterial supply to these areas. Next, leads I, aVL, V_5, and V_6 focus on the lateral (under the left armpit) side of the heart, supplied by the left circumflex artery (LCx) which branches from the left main coronary artery (LMCA). Next are leads V_1 and V_2; these leads view the septum which is fed by the septal

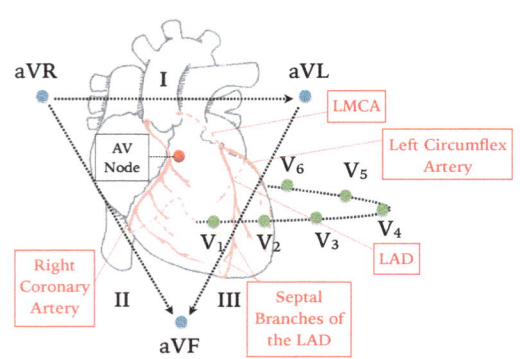

Figure 3.3: *Coronary Artery Supply in Relation to the Lead Vantages of Frontal and Horizontal Leads.*

branches of the left anterior descending artery (LAD); for the purposes of this text, knowledge that the septum is supplied by the LAD is sufficient. Finally, leads V_3 and V_4 view the anterior portion of the left ventricle, which is fed by the LAD as well. All of these regions are represented on the EKG. The attached reference sheet located at the back of the book may assist you further in visualizing these regions.

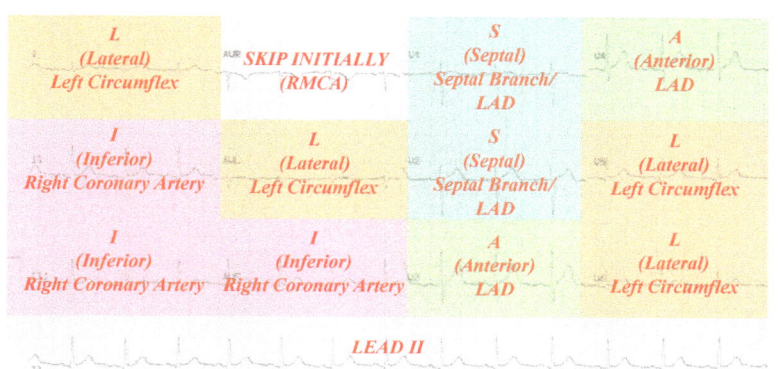

Figure 3.4: *Regional Associations Using "Lie, Lie, Sal" or "LII, LI, SSAALL." EKG from liftl.com.*

One quick-and-easy way to remember the regions of the heart on the 12-lead EKG is to remember the phrase, "Lie, Lie, Sal" or "LII, LI, SSAALL." From lead I, begin labeling this acronym downward, column by column (*figure 3.4*). Skip aVR for now; the reason for this will become apparent in subsequent sections. The representation of this labeling is L for lateral, I for inferior, S for septal, and A for anterior. Commit these primary regions and their locations to memory: inferior, lateral, septal, and anterior.

Criteria for Myocardial Infarction Diagnosis

The diagnostic criteria for a NSTEMI and STEMI are *ST change greater than two millimeters in two adjoining leads,* meaning a similar QRS elevation (STEMI) or depression (NSTEMI) in two leads viewing the same region of the heart (some sources and EMS regions specify only one millimeter change). For example, two adjoining leads that look at the lateral wall of the heart would be leads V_5 and V_6. Another pair of adjoining leads are leads II and III, which look at the inferior wall (review *figure 3.4* above). Exceptions are V_2 (septal) and V_3 (anterior) and V_4 (anterior) and V_5 (lateral), as these lead pairs are adjacent to each other on the heart surface but read different areas of the myocardium (*figure 3.5*). Infarctions read by these horizontal electrodes can involve two areas of the heart

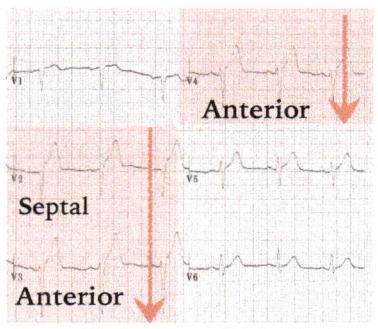

Figure 3.5: *Anteroseptal Infarction in V_2 - V_4. EKG from liftl.com.*

due to their sequential proximity and similar coronary blood flow, making it possible to have an anteroseptal (both LAD flow) and anterolateral infarct (both LMCA flow). These are common findings during a myocardial infarction, yet always first look for regional similarity. An example of a lateral STEMI with ST elevation in adjoining leads I and aVL is shown in *figure 3.6*.

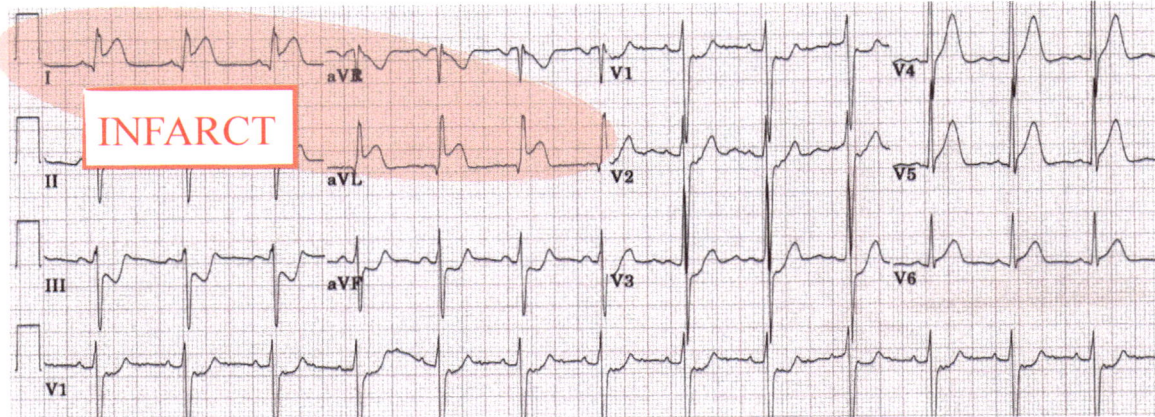

Figure 3.6: *Lateral STEMI Shown in Leads I and aVL Consistent with an Infarct to the Upper Lateral Wall of the Left Ventricle. EKG from liftl.com.*

These lateral leads are both supplied by the LCx. Note that V_5 and V_6 show minimal change; less change in V_5 and V_6, with concurrent ST elevation in leads I and aVL, assist in locating the approximate level of the occlusion within the artery or its branches because the higher the occlusion, the more area supplied a given artery will be affected (discussed later). An example of an inferior STEMI with ST elevation noted in the inferior leads II, III, and aVF:

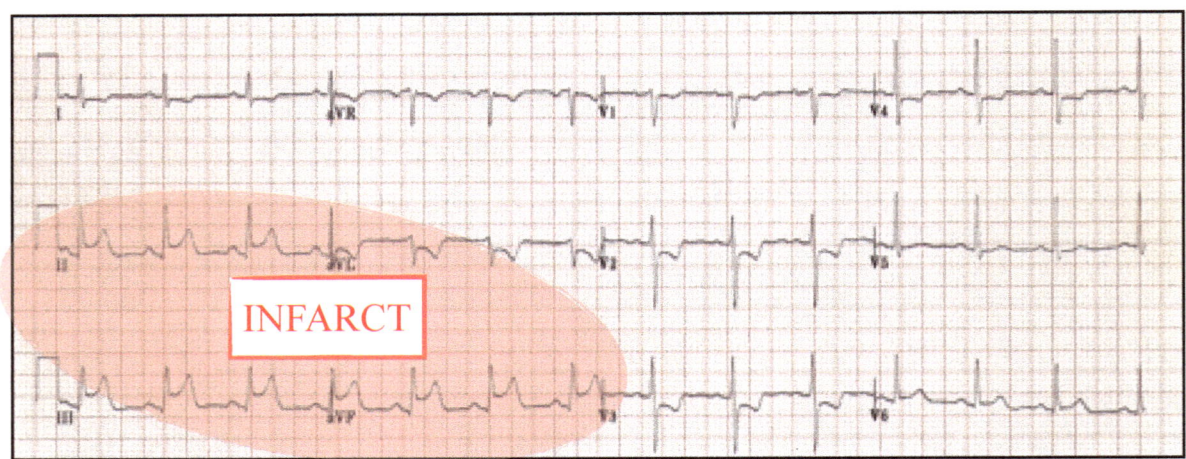

Figure 3.7: *Inferior STEMI Shown in Leads II, III, and aVL Consistent with an Occlusion of the Right Coronary Artery. EKG from liftl.com.*

Figures 3.6 and 3.7 also show **reciprocal change**, a simple yet vital concept to understand.

Reciprocal Change

During an infarct, a lack of arterial oxygen and nutrients causes damage to a specific region (or regions) of the heart, shown as ST elevation on the EKG. Should these elevations become increasingly pronounced, a mirror image can be seen on the opposite side of the heart. So, if you were to stab the area of infarction (ST elevation) with a long needle—running it straight through the heart—the region where the tip exits on the other side will reveal ST depression (*figure 3.8*). This is termed *reciprocal change*.

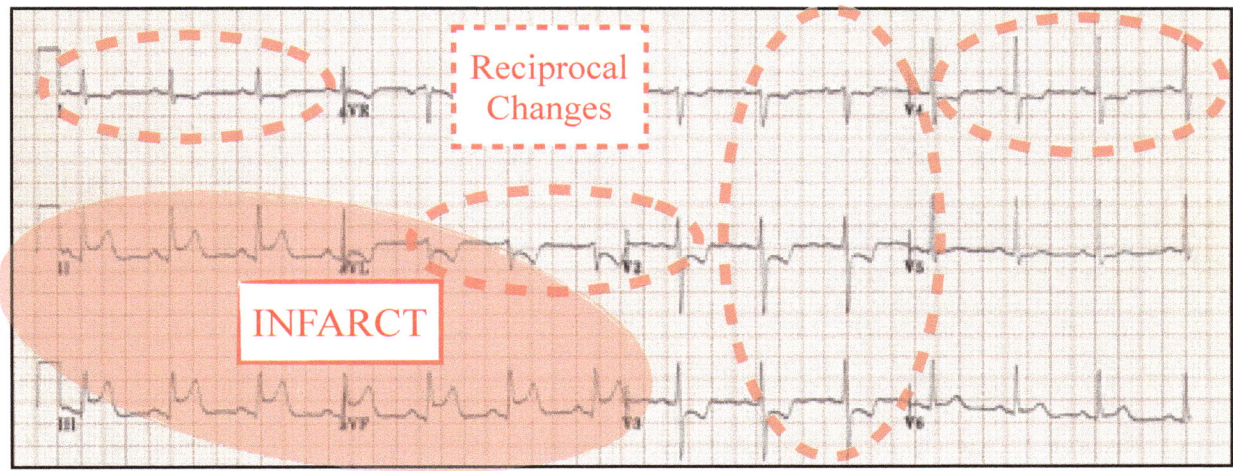

Figure 3.8: *Inferior STEMI Shown in Leads II, III, and aVL With Reciprocal Changes in the Lateral, Septal and Anterior Leads. EKG from liftl.com.*

Reciprocal change during an MI may also be caused by ischemia due to arterial insufficiency in another area of the heart. For example, think of three people rowing through a section of Class 5 rapids of the Colorado River. If one person suddenly breaks their arm on a passing branch, the other passengers must take up the slack or risk capsizing, which could be fatal. The remaining passengers must now paddle harder to keep the raft afloat, and, with time, will become fatigued. Furthermore, should these passengers be in poor physical condition for the rapids, they will tire earlier, allowing the rapids to eventually overtake them.

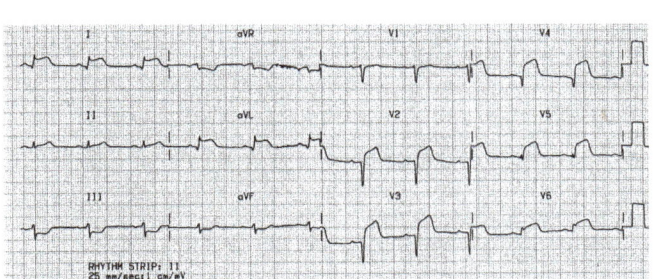

Figure 3.9: *Lateral, Anteroseptal STEMI With Reciprocal Change Inferiorly. From liftl.com.*

In short, reciprocal change is an ominous sign and is associated with worse outcomes. *Figure 3.9 (previous page)* is another example of reciprocal changes on a 12-lead EKG. Note the infarct in the lateral, septal, and anterior leads of I, aVL, and V_2 through V_6 shown by ST elevation. Reciprocal changes are noted primarily in the inferior leads III and aVF. Given what we already know about the coronary artery supply, it's apparent that this EKG is a sinister one because it reveals an occlusion to the proximal LAD and the left circumflex arteries, thus affecting the entire left side of the heart. This patient is in dire need of catheterization or thrombolytic therapy.

Lateral Infarction

Lateral infarctions occur on the left side of the heart primarily due to an occlusion of the LCx or one of its branches. The lateral heart surface is best viewed by leads I, aVL, V_5 and V_6, as these leads look leftward from the AV node (*yellow arrows, figure 3.10*). Depending on the location of the thrombus within the LCx, differing lateral leads will reveal ST change; for example, leads I and aVL reveal higher

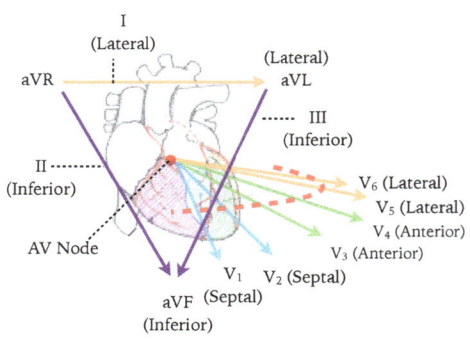

Figure 3.10: *Diagram Showing the Leftward Vantage of the Lateral Leads I, aVL, V_5 and V_6.*

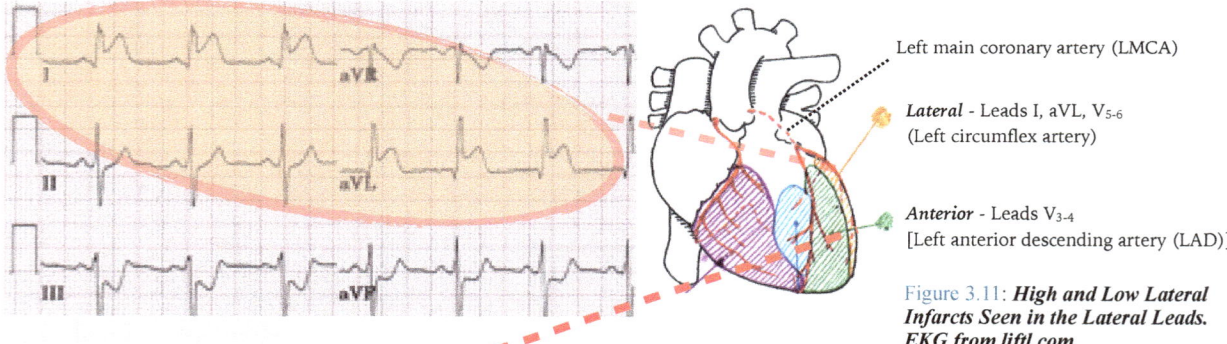

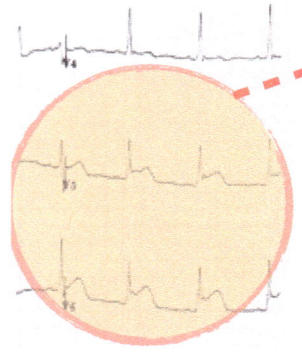

Figure 3.11: *High and Low Lateral Infarcts Seen in the Lateral Leads. EKG from liftl.com.*

occlusions, likely due to a branch of the proximal LCx, whereas leads V_5 and V_6 reveal lower occlusions due to their position below the vantage of leads I and aVL. *Figure 3.11* provides examples of occlusions of the lateral heart surface: one involving the proximal LCx, the other, distal. Be sure to note the reciprocal changes in the inferior leads III and aVF as well.

It's not uncommon for lateral injuries to have anterior involvement due to the anatomy of the coronary artery system. The LCx branches from the LMCA, as does the LAD which supplies the anterior and septal portions of the heart (figure 3.12). Therefore, the higher the infarct, the more likely the entire LAD will be involved and possibly the LMCA itself, resulting in total ischemia of the left ventricle. Figure 3.13 is another example of a high lateral infarct shown primarily in leads I and aVL.

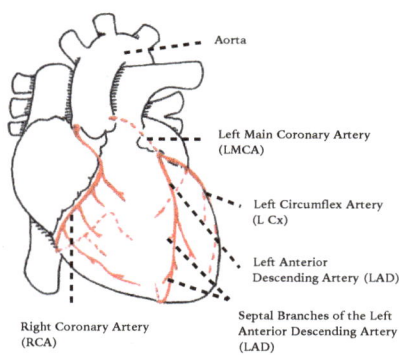

Figure 3.12: *Coronary Artery Anatomy of the Heart.*

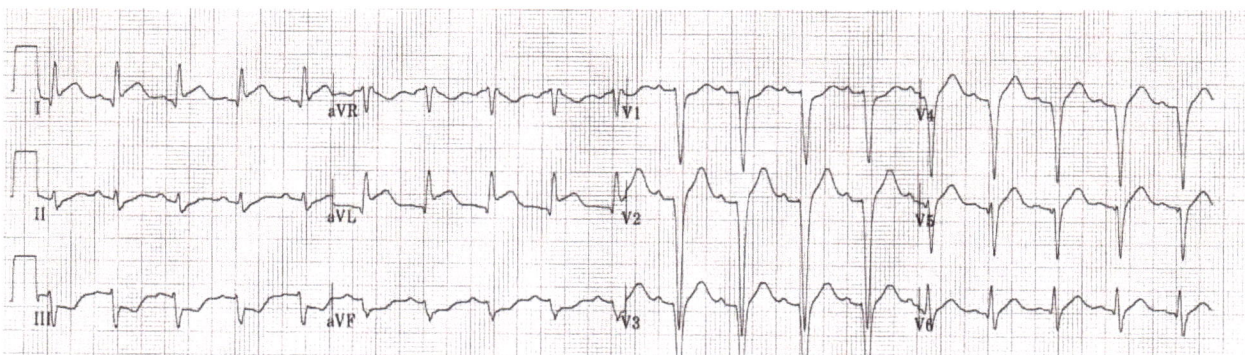

Figure 3.13: *High Lateral Infarct Shown by ST-elevation in the Lateral Leads I and aVL. From liftl.com.*

Note the ST elevations in leads I and aVL with reciprocal changes in the inferior leads II, III, and aVF. There are no clear findings in leads V_5 and V_6, making the occlusion likely within a higher branch of the left circumflex artery.

Inferior Infarction

Inferior infarctions account for nearly half of all STEMIs, yet have a slightly higher survival rate than other MIs. Prolonged infarctions within the inferior aspect of the heart are often the cause of bradyarrhythmias, including 2nd- and 3rd-degree heart blocks.

Inferior infarcts effect the bottom, and

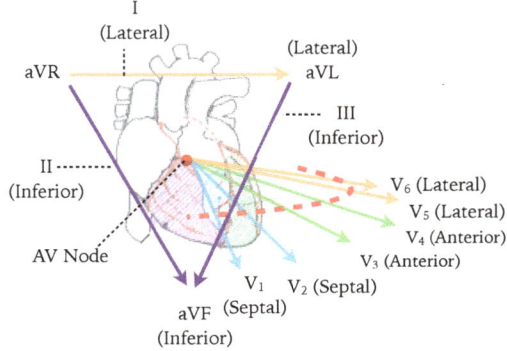

Figure 3.14: *Diagram Showing the Rightward and Bottom Vantages of the Inferior Leads II, III, and aVF (Purple).*

occasionally, the right and posterior portions of the heart. They're caused by an occlusion involving either the RCA or one of its branches. Leads II, III, and aVF identify inferior infarctions due to their vantage [*figure 3.14 (previous page) and 3.15*]. The location of the occlusion within the RCA is essential to understand, for the more proximal the occlusion, the more likely the right ventricle is involved and a right-sided infarction has occurred. Knowledge of this phenomenon is critical, for diagnosis and treatment of a right ventricular infarct differs from other infarctions (discussed later in the chapter).

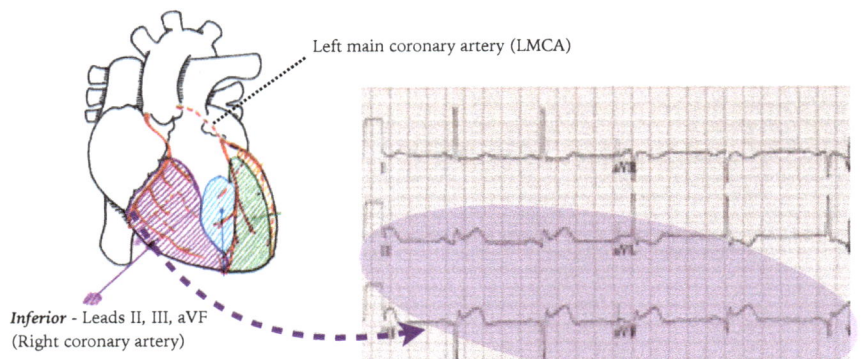

Figure 3.15: *Diagram Showing the Inferior Heart and the Right Coronary Artery with a STEMI in Leads II, III, and aVF. EKG from liftl.com.*

Inferior infarcts are associated with posterior infarcts as well, as the RCA tracks along the inferior portion to the back of the heart. Be aware that signs of a posterior infarct may accompany inferior findings, further revealing the volatility of the patients' condition. We'll discuss posterior infarcts in an upcoming section. *Figure 3.16* is an example of an inferior infarct as shown in leads II, III, and aVF, with posterior concerns in V_{1-2}:

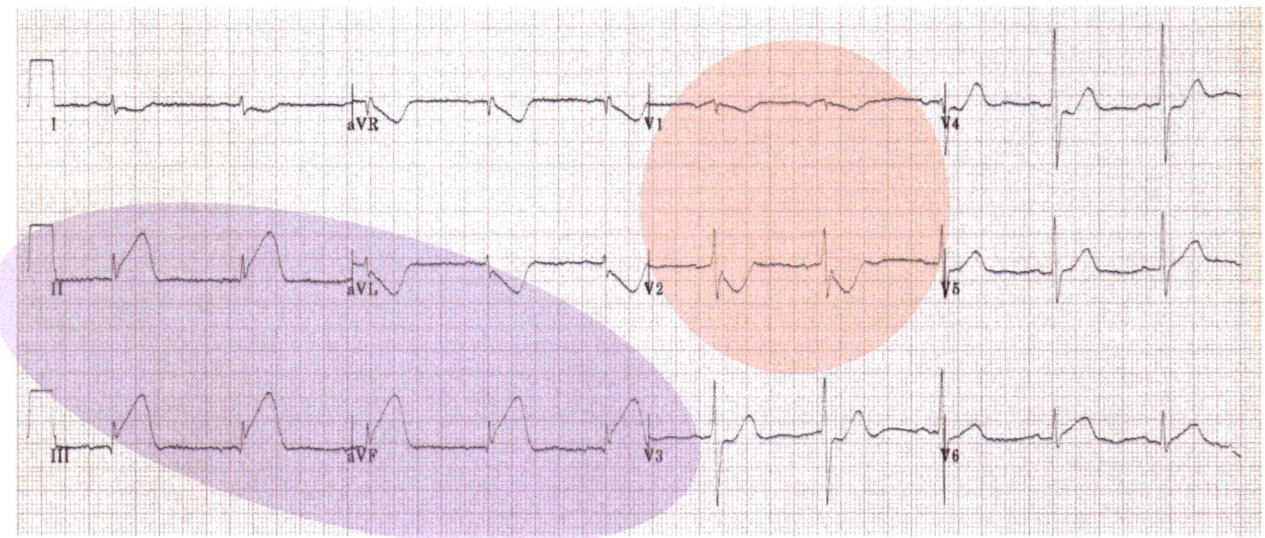

Figure 3.16: *Inferior STEMI Revealed in Leads II, III, and aVF with Reciprocal Changes in the Septal Leads V_1 and V_2 Concerning for Posterior Infarction. EKG from liftl.com.*

Again, note the reciprocal changes in the lateral, septal, and anterior leads. These changes indicate the level of stress the heart is experiencing and are a concern for potential posterior involvement (Discussed later).

Septal and Anterior Infarctions

Septal and anterior infarctions have a higher mortality rate than other infarctions, and often cause new-onset left bundle-branch blocks (Wilner, B; de Lemos, J.A., et al., 2017). These infarctions commonly have a diffuse pattern that cross horizontal leads V_2 and V_3 (*figure 3.17*).

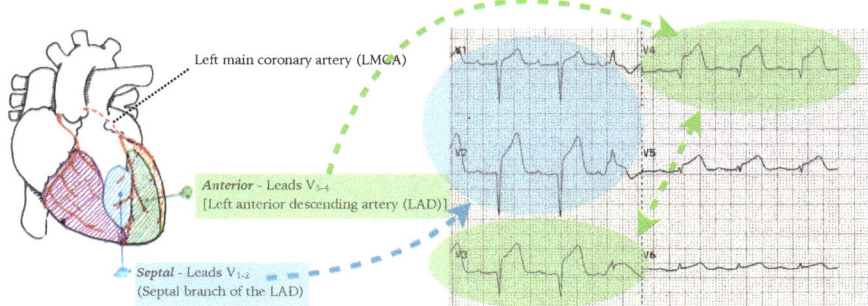

Figure 3.17: *Septal and Anterior STEMI Revealed in Leads V_{1-4} with Lateral Involvement. EKG from liftl.com.*

Anterior infarctions result from an occlusion of the LAD, while septal infarctions are brought about by occlusions of one of the lower septal branches of the LAD.

A higher occlusion of the LAD will show changes in both the septal leads V_1-V_2 and anterior leads V_3-V_4 (*figure 3.18*). The higher the LAD occlusion, the higher the mortality rate. A complete restriction of the LAD is often termed a "Widow Maker" due to its high mortality rate caused by reduced oxygenation to such a large portion of the left ventricle.

Septal infarctions are revealed in leads V_1-V_2. While rare, septal infarctions result from a blockage of one of the septal branches of the LAD. Furthermore, ST segment depression in leads V_1-V_2 is highly suspicious for a posterior infarction, as these findings may be the result of reciprocal changes opposite of the septal leads on the posterior myocardium. Posterior MIs are reviewed in the following section.

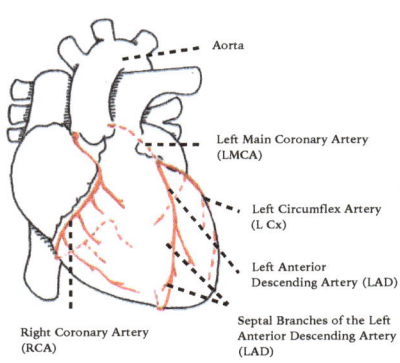

Figure 3.18: Basic Coronary Artery Representation Revealing the Left Anterior Descending and Its Septal Branches.

Other Infarctions

An astute prehospital provider is aware of three additional infarcts that are not readily apparent: they are the right ventricular, or right-sided MI; the posterior MI; and the complete LMCA MI. These infarctions are important for their peculiarities: right-sided MIs require a slight deviation in treatment, while posterior MIs often appear as a NSTEMI, making it easy to miss the reciprocal injury to detrimental effect. Finally, LMCA infarctions can be subtle, but effect such a large portion of the left ventricle that they quickly lead to instability and cardiac arrest, prompting the need for situational readiness and rapid transport should the patient decompensate. The ability to identify these three infarctions is essential to providing prompt and appropriate care.

Right Ventricular Myocardial Infarction

Right-sided MIs are relatively easy to identify. They are the result of an occlusion of the RCA. As discussed earlier, occlusion to the RCA causes acute ST elevation in inferior leads II, III, and aVF, and indicates an inferior infarction, yet, depending on the exact site of the occlusion, supply to the right ventricle may be cut off as well. Consequently, an inferior infarction often veils right-sided involvement.

Identification of a Right Ventricular Myocardial Infarction

A right-sided STEMI is verified by removing the V_4 electrode and placing it on the right breast at precisely the same location as the left (*figure 3.19*). If ST elevation is seen in this new lead, termed V_4R ("R" for "right"), the diagnosis is confirmed. Because of the electrodes new position away from the standard AV impulse deflection toward lead II, the deflection of the QRS in V_4R will be negative as the impulse is now traveling away from this lead. Looking at a cross-section of the top of the heart provides a good illustration (*figure 3.20, next page*). Once placement has been achieved, STEMI identification is reasonably straightforward. It is important to identify

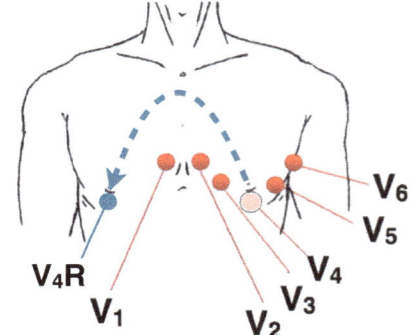

Figure 3.19: *V_4R Placement for Right Ventricular Infarct Identification.*

Diagnostic Criteria

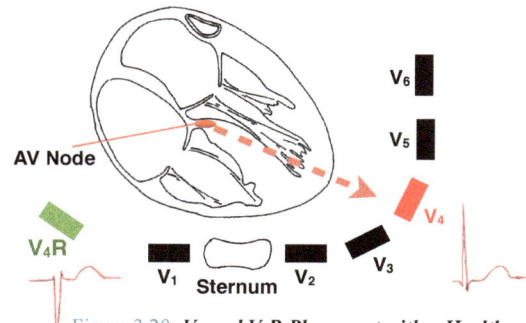

Figure 3.20: *V_4 and V_4R Placement with a Healthy Precordial Axis and Corresponding QRS complexes.*

which lead is V_4R by labeling it on the printout as in *figure 3.21*. Note the negative deflection of V_4R compared to the naturally placed precordial leads of V_{3-6}.

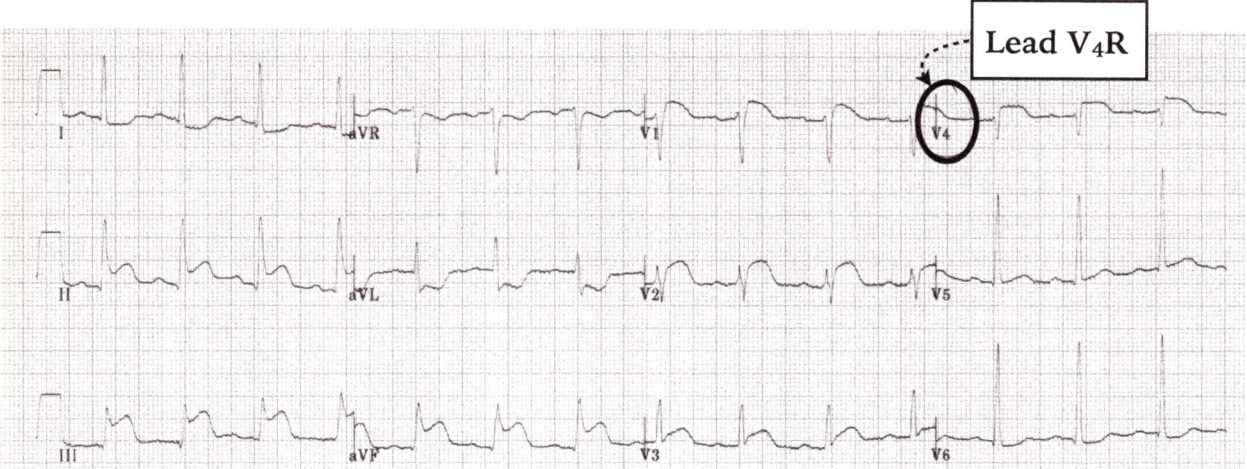

Figure 3.21: *Inferior STEMI with Right Sided EKG Revealing ST Elevation in V_4R. Note the Anteroseptal Changes as Well. EKG from liftl.com.*

Treatment of a Right Ventricular Infarction

Because the right ventricle is very sensitive to preload, and since nitrites reduce preload and cardiac output, nitroglycerin given to a patient with a right-ventricular infarction can severely drop blood pressure, leading to rapid decompensation. It's like attempting to blow water through a straw while you're out of breath and then suddenly the diameter of the straw is increased significantly, making your job even harder. There are two ways to address a right-sided MI, depending on your local protocols.

First and foremost, never administer nitroglycerin to a patient with an inferior STEMI until a right ventricular infarction is either ruled out or considered. Once right ventricular changes are confirmed, it's imperative to either give a 500 milliliter bolus of normal saline to the patient before nitroglycerin, or the nitroglycerin is withheld altogether. Other approaches include giving a 500 milliliter bolus to any inferior MI before nitroglycerin administration without V_4R confirmation, unless contraindications exists. This approach both saves time and decreases patient risk. Finally, if your course of action is unsure, it is always appropriate to contact the hospital for physician direction with any inferior infarction before nitroglycerin administration.

Overlooking a right-sided MI is easy, and because a rapid reduction in preload to a stressed heart can have serious implications, suspicion should be high with any inferior infarction. The incidence of a right ventricle MI associated with an inferior STEMI is 30-50% (Jeffers and Parks, 2019); therefore, if a right ventricle infarction is suspected, *always* bolus or rule out the diagnosis of right-sided involvement via V$_4$R before the administration of nitrites.

Posterior Myocardial infarction

Posterior MIs are often missed or overlooked in the sphere of prehospital medicine. They're not a common occurrence and present with findings that are often subtle, requiring sound clinical recognition skills.

Identification of a Posterior Infarction

Posterior MIs involve the posterior surface of the heart where the standard 12-lead EKG does not read (unless you work in a region that utilizes a 15-lead monitor). Because this area is not routinely assessed by the standard EKG, a posterior injury will present with reciprocal findings of ischemia and mild AV deflection changes in the septal (V$_1$,V$_2$), and anterior leads (V$_3$,V$_4$), opposite of the infarction. These findings commonly go unrecognized or are attributed to a NSTEMI, unless the prehospital provider has the knowledge of posterior MI presentation on the 12-lead EKG.

Looking at a cross-section of the top of the heart, one can appreciate how the morphology changes during a posterior MI (*figure 3.22*). As damage occurs in the posterior region of the myocardium, it becomes more

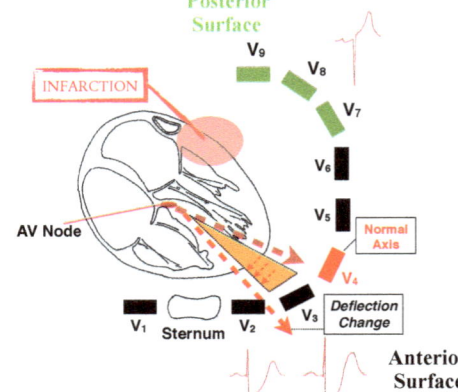

Figure 3.22: *Transverse Plane of the Heart Depicting the Horizontal Axis Shift Caused by Posterior Myocardial Injury.*

difficult for conduction to pass, resulting in a progressive horizontal axis shift toward the septum, away from the injured tissues. When this occurs, the septal (V_1, V_2), in which the QRS should have a primarily negative deflection in a healthy heart, becomes increasingly positive as the impulse shifts toward the positive electrodes of these leads. Concurrently, as the infarct progresses, reciprocal ischemic changes are seen in the septal (V_1, V_2) and anterior leads (V_3, V_4) as well, as these areas attempt to compensate for the damaged posterior muscle (*figure 3.23*). While the ischemia is obvious to EMS

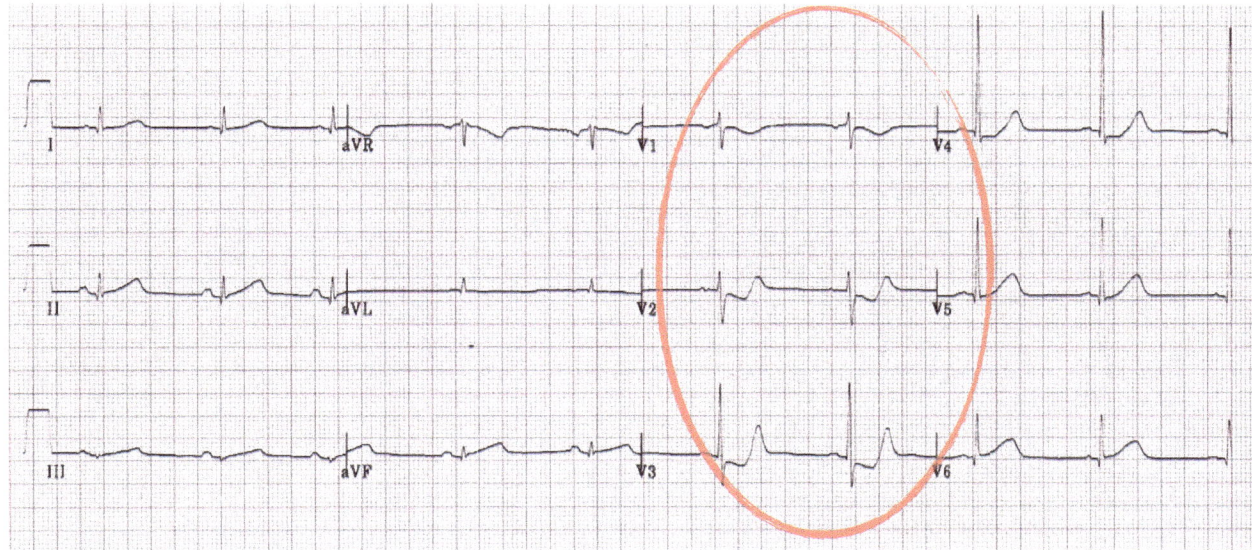

Figure 3.23: *EKG Suggestive of a Posterior Infarction as Shown by Increased Septal Amplitude of the R Wave and ST Depression in the Septal and Anterior Leads. EKG from liftl.com.*

personnel, the potential for reciprocal change is missed, which is why it is often seen as a NSTEMI pattern when, in actuality, it is a STEMI.

How to Assess the Posterior Heart Surface

Confirmation of a posterior MI requires repositioning of the horizontal leads, yet instead of one lead, as in a right-ventricular infarction, three are moved. A pearl to take away from this is that repositioning of the leads is time-dependent; If the patient is not stable or the diagnosis is obvious, forego these steps.

To confirm a posterior MI, relocate leads V_{4-6} to the patient's back, lateral to the spine on the left side. Once in position, these leads become leads V_{7-9}; V_4 becomes V_7, V_5 becomes V_8, V_6 becomes V_9. Landmarks are quite easy to find. V_8 should be placed just

Diagnostic Criteria

below the inferior angle of the scapula with V_7 and V_9 affixed just left and right of V_8, approximately 1/2 to 3/4 inches apart (figure 3.24). Because of this placement, the deflection of the QRS on the printout will now be negative, with the exception of any ST elevation (figure 3.25). Be sure to indicate which leads are posterior on the printout to avoid confusion as to which printout is which.

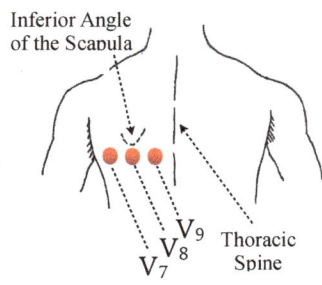

Figure 3.24: *Posterior Placement of Leads V_{7-9}.*

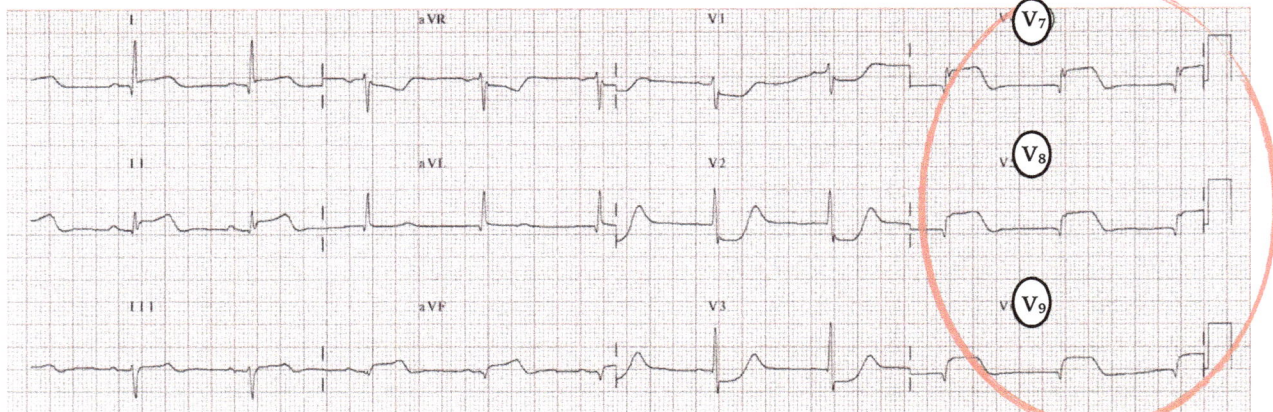

Figure 3.25: *Inferior and Posterior Myocardial Injury as Shown in Leads II, III, aVF, and V_{7-9}. EKG from liftl.com.*

Left Main Coronary Artery (LMCA) Myocardial Infarction

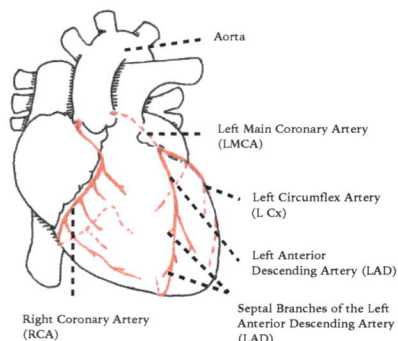

Figure 3.26: Basic Coronary Artery Representation Revealing the Left Anterior Descending and Its Septal Branches.

LMCA infarctions are nasty, as they affect the entire left side of the myocardium. Understanding the arterial flow of the heart is vital in identifying a LMCA occlusion (figure 3.26), for these patients have a higher probability of arresting during transport.

As explained earlier, leads I, aVL, and V_{1-6} are all supplied by the LMCA and its branches. Lower infarcts in any of the branches of the LMCA, such as the septal branch of the LAD (V_1, V_2), the LAD itself (V_3, V_4), or the LCx (I, aVL, V_5, V_6) will reveal ST changes in the specific regions they supply. However, should the occlusion occur higher within the LMCA itself, before the LAD or LCx branch bifurcates, all or most the left ventricular leads (I, aVL, and V_{1-6}) will reveal ischemic changes. These findings are an ominous sign. *Figure 3.27* is an example of how a LMCA infarction can appear on a prehospital EKG:

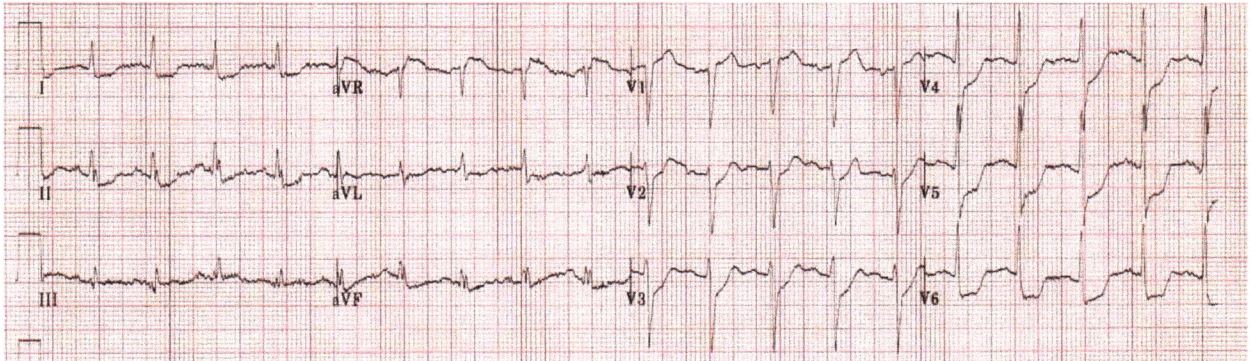

Figure 3.27: **ST Depression Shown Diffusely Across the Entire Precordium (V_{1-6}), Including the High Lateral Leads I and aVL. From liftl.com.**

Note the ST elevation in lead aVR and diffuse precordial ischemia (*figure 3.28*). While aVR is initially overlooked, it can be the only indicator of an early LMCA infarct. The concept of an LMCA infarct causes difficulty because aVR has no adjoining lead, therefore there's no comparison as with the paired leads. Some sources note the lack of specificity in the findings of ST elevation in aVR, yet it should be considered in the prehospital realm, especially with diffuse findings of elevation or depression within the precordial leads.

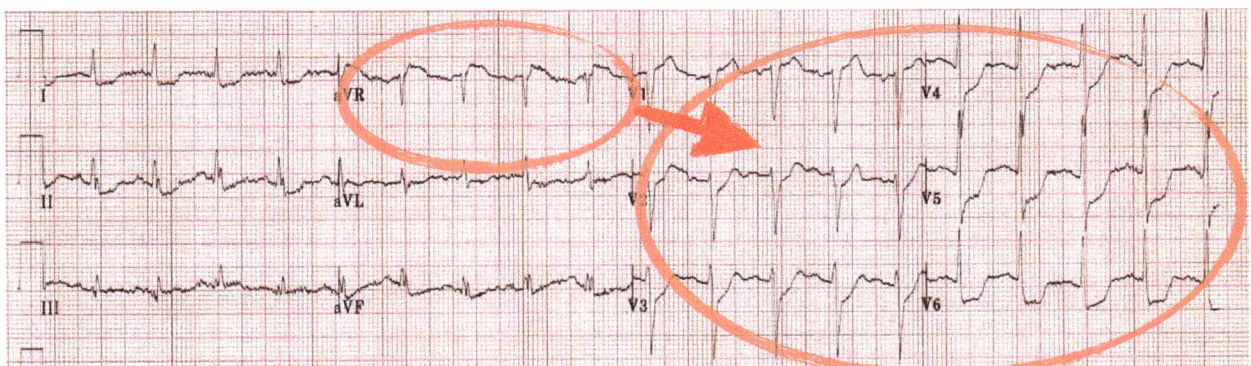

Figure 3.28: **ST Elevation Shown in aVR with Reciprocal ST Depression in the Horizontal Leads Indicating a Likely Occlusion of the Left Main Coronary Artery. EKG from liftl.com.**

This chapter contained a substantial amount of information, from coronary artery supply to diagnostic criteria of an MI, to less frequent yet significant findings. It's essential that prehospital providers understand the diagnostic criteria for an MI as well as the particular circumstances for a right-sided and posterior infarction. These two infarctions are compulsory for prehospital providers to know and identify for both treatment decisions and acuity reasons. Inability to identify any of the 12-lead EKG patterns presented within this chapter can have detrimental consequences on patient mortality.

Takeaway Notes from Chapter 3:

- *The definition of an STEMI is ST elevation greater than one to two millimeters in two leads viewing the same region (depending on your local protocols), with the exception of V_2-V_3 and V_4-V_5 as these infarctions can overlap as a result of the close proximity these electrodes have to one another.*

- *Reciprocal change is an ominous sign on the EKG.*

- *Consider right-sided MIs with all inferior infarcts and administer a 500ml bolus before any nitroglycerin administration, unless contraindicated. Consider a right-sided EKG with V_4R, time permitting.*

- *Always consider a posterior MI with ST depression in V_{1-2}, especially with an associated increase in positive QRS amplitude within these leads.*

- ***NEVER*** *delay transport to obtain a 12-lead EKG when the patient is unstable or the diagnosis is clear based off the patient's presentation and your physical exam.*

4

Cardiac Axis and Blocks For EMS

Cardiac axis is a topic dreaded by most of the students I teach. While the topic can be confusing, cardiac axis is quite simple to determine if you practice and understand the vantage points of the various leads. EMS providers don't rely heavily on axis for diagnostic purposes, yet there are a few situations where a basic understanding of this material is of use, if even for future understanding of advanced topics not covered in this text.

What is Cardiac Axis?

Cardiac axis (or more specifically ventricular axis) is the representation of the angle of depolarization as the electrical impulse leaves the AV node and travels through the conduction pathways of the ventricles. Essentially, cardiac axis is which positive electrode of a given lead the electrical impulse is aiming toward as it leaves the AV node (i.e., lead I, II, III, etc.); the trajectory of this impulse is assessed as either normal, left shift, or right shift.

Normal wiring pathways located within the cardiac muscle give preference to the larger left ventricle in a healthy individual. Any change in the direction of the current—often caused by tissue damage, increased muscle wall thickness, arrhythmia, etc—decreases conduction to the left ventricle, thus weakening its capacity to pump effectively. Cardiac axis is important concept because as the AV impulse moves further away from its normal path, left ventricular contraction strength decreases, making arrhythmias more likely and circulation less efficient.

Textbook cardiac axis is defined as and impulse leaving the AV node at an angle between -30 and +120 degrees, with 0 degrees fixed at the left armpit and +60 degrees at the left hip. For field application, this is an AV impulse

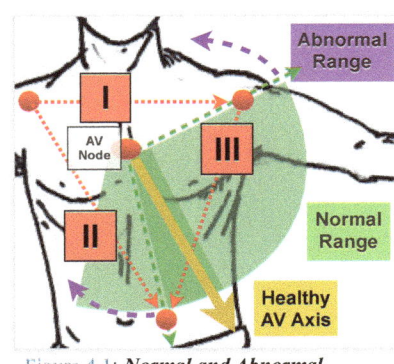

Figure 4.1: *Normal and Abnormal, Anatomic Cardiac Axis Ranges.*

traveling anywhere between the left shoulder and right hip (*figure 4.1, previous page*). Consider anything outside of this area as abnormal, as it significantly pulls conduction away from the left ventricle.

QRS Deflection and Impulse Trajectory

An increase or decrease in stimulation is represented on an EKG by the height of the QRS in a given positive electrode of a frontal lead (primarily leads I, II, and III). A positive electrode will either increase or decrease in QRS amplitude (become taller or shorter) depending on its proximity to the impulse direction leaving the AV node (*figure 4.2*). The taller the QRS in a given lead, the more the AV impulse is traveling toward it. Remember, for the purposes of EMS application, cardiac axis focuses on the frontal leads only. The following section provides some examples.

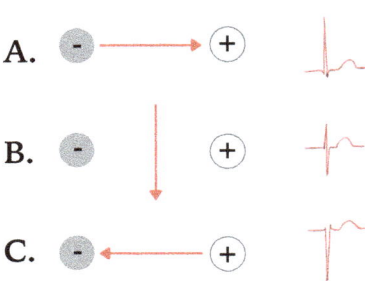

Figure 4.2: *QRS Amplitude Based on the Direction of AV Impulse to a Given Positive or Negative Electrode. A. Upright QRS due to Deflection in line with the Positive Electrode of a given Lead; B. QRS with an Impulse Traveling Equidistant to a Positive and Negative Electrode of a Given Lead; C. QRS with an Impulse Traveling Away from the Positive Electrode of a Given Lead.*

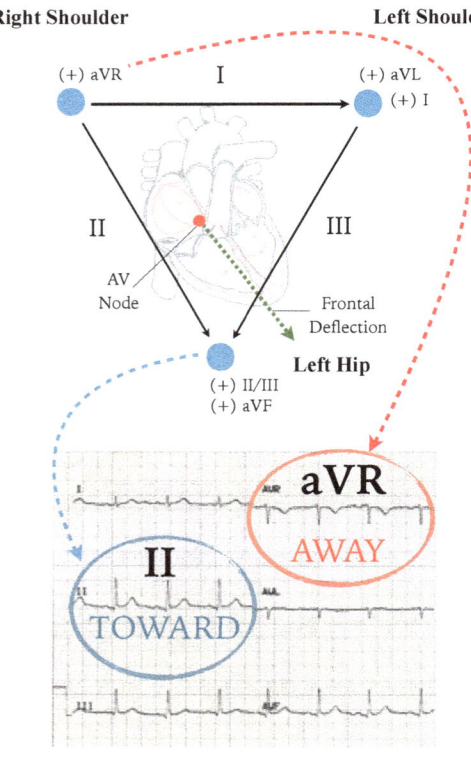

Figure 4.3: *Frontal leads of a 12-Lead EKG Revealing a Normal QRS Axis.*

Determining Cardiac Axis in the Prehospital Setting

Figure 4.3 shows the AV impulse traveling in a direction consistent with the positive electrode of lead II or the left hip, revealing adequate left ventricular stimulation. While leads I and III are also positive, they show a smaller positive QRS complex as the impulse is *less* in the path of these electrodes. Remember the statement *in the path*. This is why lead I is the smallest because it's positive electrode is further away from the path of conduction when compared to the positive electrodes of leads II and III.

You could go one step further to confirm this. If the AV impulse is traveling directly toward lead II, what lead should it be traveling away from? If the impulse is heading for the left hip (lead II), this means that it's traveling away from the right shoulder or lead aVR. Therefore, if lead II is the most positive, aVR must be negative, because conduction is traveling *away* from its positive electrode. Leads II and aVR are routinely found on the bottom of many 12-lead EKG printouts for determining cardiac axis. Though exact angles are not important for prehospital providers, this method of quick comparison confirms a normal axis between -30 and +120 degrees.

As shown, the concept of cardiac axis is simple if the vantages of positive electrodes on the frontal leads are understood. Remember that leads II and aVF receive impulses at roughly the left hip and leads I and aVL receive at the left shoulder. The aVR lead (positive at the right shoulder) is in a league of its own. aVR should never be positive unless the electrodes are misplaced or there's a significant axis shift toward the right shoulder. Should the axis deviate toward the right shoulder, leads I, II, and III will all be negative.

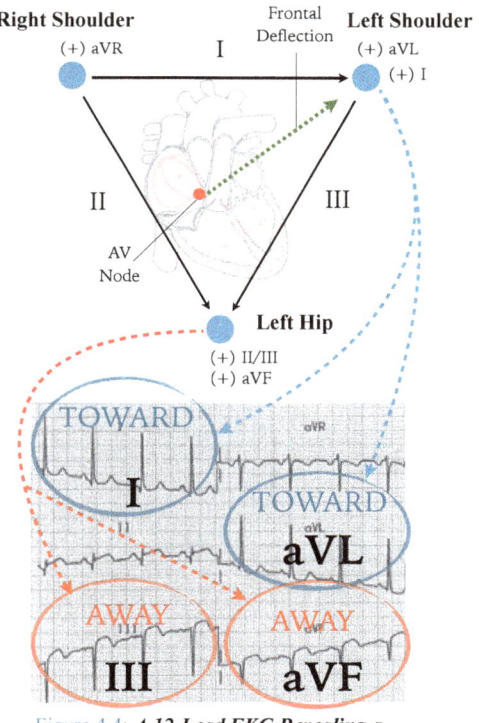

Figure 4.4: *A 12-Lead EKG Revealing a Leftward Axis Deviation.*

In some cases, it's difficult to ascertain which lead is more positive. For example, in *figure 4.4*, it appears that both lead I and aVL are equally positive; this similarity indicates the AV impulse is traveling toward these leads, and, because I and aVL are positive at the left shoulder, an impulse traveling equally toward each will represent as an upright QRS complex in both leads on the EKG. This is confirmed by viewing a positive lead that's opposite the left shoulder, such as lead III or aVF. Note lead III and aVF are both negative. This method confirms a leftward deflection of the impulse from the AV node that's greater than -30 degrees, and it's termed a *leftward axis shift*.

In contrast, a *right axis shift* is an AV impulse deviation toward the right shoulder. As a result, the positive electrodes of leads III and aVR will become increasingly positive, while the positive of the left shoulder (I, aVL) will become negative (*figure 4.5*). With practice this concept is useful for prehospital diagnostics.

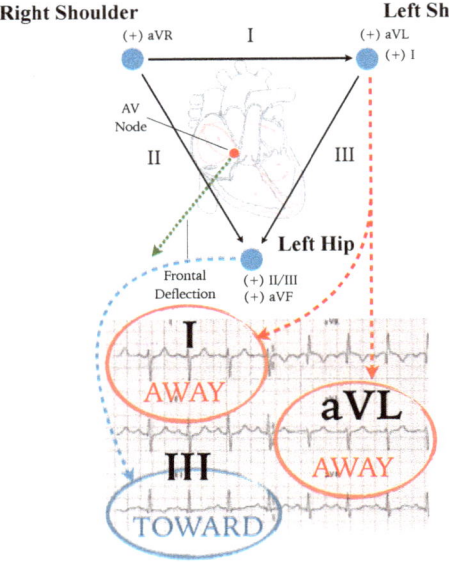

Figure 4.5: *A 12-Lead EKG Revealing a Rightward Axis Deviation.*

Cardiac Axis for EMS

For the purposes of EMS, the easiest way to determine axis is to simply look at all of the frontal leads on the EKG. Which is the most positive? If lead II is the most positive and aVR is negative, you are done, as the axis is within the normal range. Another method is to look at leads I, II, and III, if they're all positive, the axis is in the normal range of -30° to +120°. It's always a good idea to glance at aVR, for this lead should *always* have a negative deflection, unless there's a major axis shift toward the right shoulder, or a lead is misplaced.

As the AV impulse moves toward the left (leads I and aVL), or right (leads III and aVR), the positive amplitude of the QRS within these leads will increase, as they're receiving more conduction. Think of knob on a radio (*figure 4.6*). As you switch channels from right to left and vis-versa, you're increasing input to one channel while decreasing to another. This concept is the same with cardiac axis: as you increase the current toward a positive electrode of a given lead, you simultaneously decrease it to its inverse.

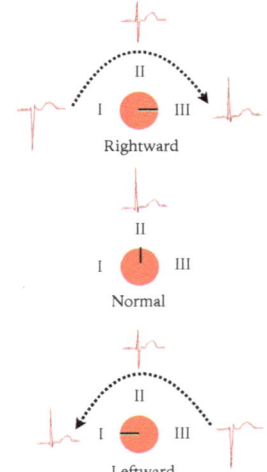

Further simplifying axis shift, we can add two small notations to the EKG in order to aid in axis determination if it appears abnormal on first glance. If leads I, II and III do not all contain positive QRS complexes, label aVR "right" (R=right) and aVL "left" (L=left) (*figure 4.7 and 4.8, next page*); whichever lead has a positive QRS complex is the axis shift, right or left. For example, if aVR is positive, then it is a right shift; if aVL is positive, left

Figure 4.6: *Knob Diagram Showing the Effects of Increased Positivity or Negativity to a Given Lead on the Right or Left Side of the Heart.*

shift. Again, this only applies when the deflection of leads I, II, and III vary is amplitude, and the electrodes are properly placed.

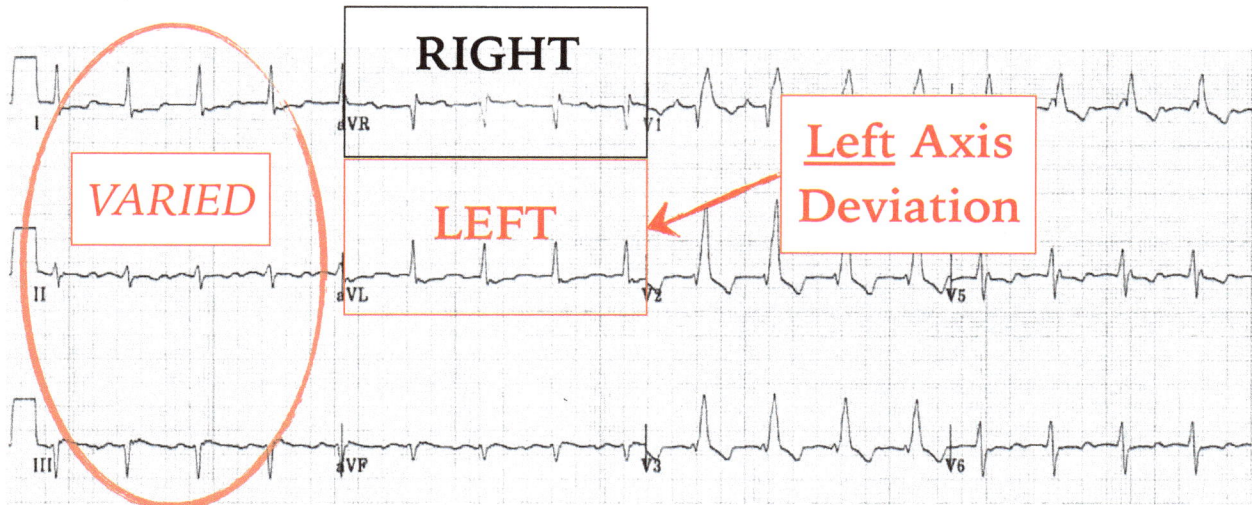

Figure 4.7: *A 12-Lead EKG Revealing a Leftward Axis Deviation.*

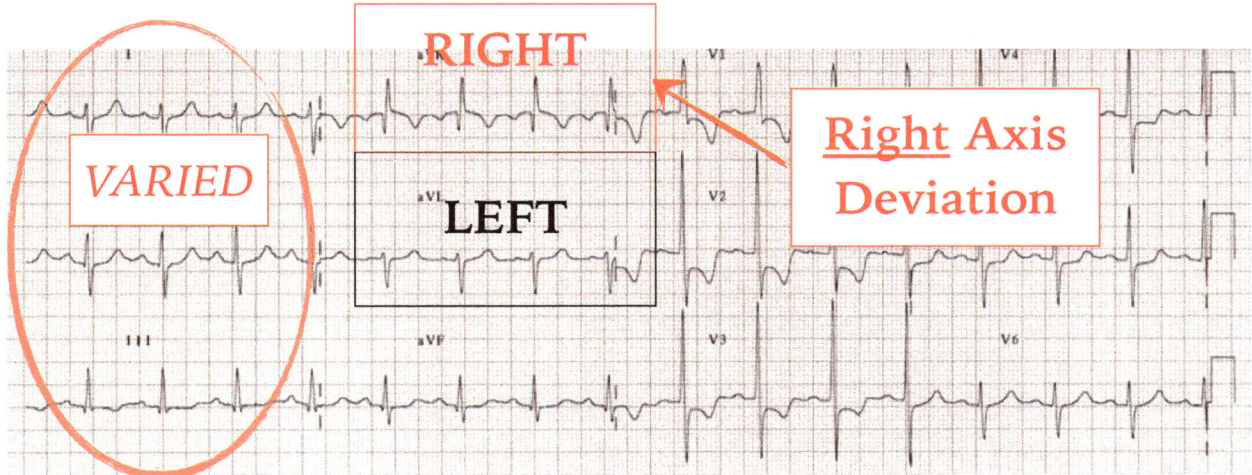

Figure 4.8: *A 12-Lead EKG Revealing a Rightward Axis Deviation.*

So why is this important for EMS? Structural changes, such as a tissue loss during an MI, can alter the normal conduction pathways of the heart by slowing, shifting, or blocking the AV impulse. Furthermore, it can clue you into the existence of underlying cardiac co-morbidities and assist in identification of a left bundle branch block (LBBB), which—in a patient without a known cardiac history—is suspicious for an underlying MI in these cases.

Left Bundle Branch Blocks in the Prehospital Venue

While right bundle blocks (RBBB) do have their significance, they have little application in the prehospital setting. Left bundle branch blocks (LBBB), however, are more concerning as they occasionally result from an underlying anterior or anteroseptal infarction. While diagnosis of an acute MI in the presence of a LBBB is difficult to diagnose, especially in the prehospital setting, paramedics should be suspicious of a coronary event in patients without known cardiac history, yet with positive cardiac symptoms and a LBBB on the EKG. Sgarbossa criteria is not discussed in this text.

Although it's not necessarily recommended that a LBBB be given STEMI activation, transport to a cardiac center may be warranted. Studies have shown only 2-4% of chest pain patients with a new onset of LBBB have an occlusion. Despite the low probability, transporting suspected cardiac patients to the appropriate facility based on your signs, symptoms, and clinical judgement is never wrong because your patient with a LBBB may be within that 2-4%. Prehospital providers don't have access to the many tools available within the hospital, yet do have ample time for a patient to decompensate. Moving patients toward facilities that treat cardiac pathologies when the symptoms suggest such a cause, whether an obvious STEMI or not, is always appropriate.

Field Diagnosis of a Left Bundle Branch Block

Recall that the normal QRS width is less than 1.2 millimeters (*figure 4.9*). In the case of a RBBB or LBBB, this width increases due to a reversal and delay in septal depolarization, whether by an acute coronary event or chronic conditions. With a LBBB, septal depolarization is interrupted, causing a delay in conduction toward the left ventricle.

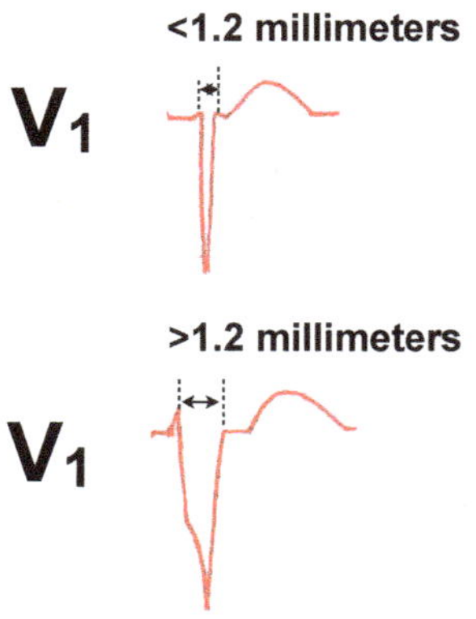

Figure 4.9: *Normal vs. Widened QRS Width Indicating the Potential for a Bundle Branch Block.*

Field diagnosis of a LBBB is not difficult. Scanning your 12-lead EKG printout, the QRS complex will present with a width greater than 1.2 millimeters across all leads on the printout. Once this widening is identified, look at lead V_1 (*figure 4.10*). Since a bundle branch block represents

Cardiac Axis

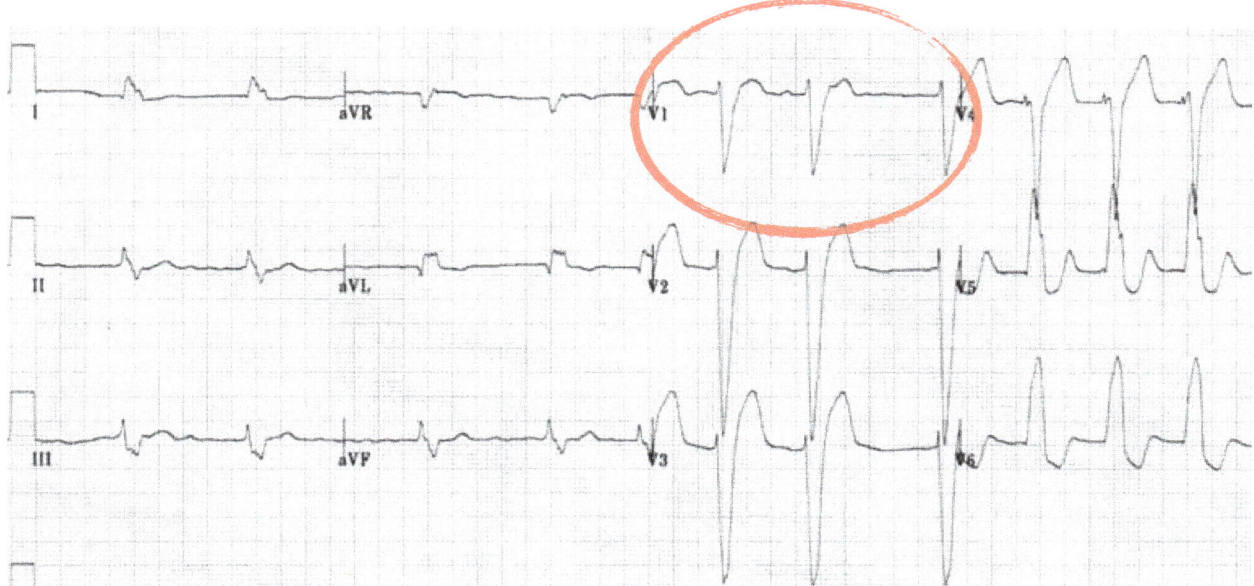

Figure 4.10: **LBBB on 12-Lead with Concentration on the Septal Lead V_1 for Diagnosis.**

abnormal depolarization within the septum of the heart, it only makes sense to focus on a lead that records electrical activity through the septum, such as V_1. Looking at V_1,

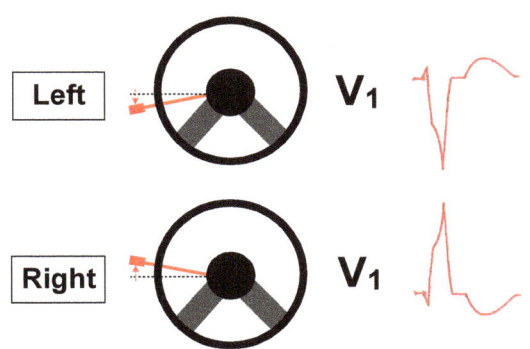

Figure 4.11: **Turn Signal Diagram to Aid in Determining Left vs. Right Bundle Branch Blocks.**

there's a trick to determine a RBBB verses LBBB. While not 100% diagnostic, it's perfect for field personnel.

Think of the turn signal on the steering column of your car (*figure 4.11*). If you flip the signal lever down, you wish to turn left; flip the lever up for right. That's the memory trick: if the QRS deflection of lead V_1 is below the isoelectric line in the presence of a widened QRS, it's likely a LBBB (the lever is flipped down, left turn); if the QRS of V_1 is above the isoelectric line, it's likely a RBBB (the lever is flipped up, right turn). Easy. Finally, there's a matter of axis deviation; LBBBs are associated with a left axis shift.

Quick review of prehospital criteria for a LBBB:

1. QRS width >1.2 millimeters across all leads.
2. Downward QRS deflection in V_1 (Upward deflection in RBBB).
3. Leftward axis as seen in I and aVL.

Figure 4.12 is an example of a LBBB meeting this criteria on the 12-lead EKG:

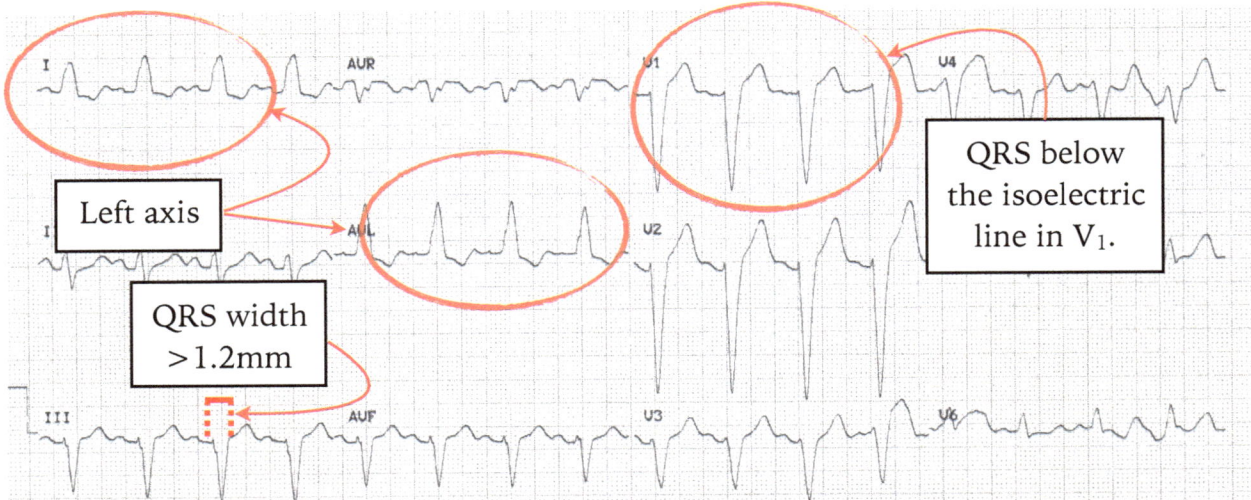

Figure 4.12: *12-Lead EKG Revealing Criteria for a Left Bundle Branch Block.*

As discussed earlier, there are only a few practical scenarios where cardiac axis determination applies in the prehospital setting, yet it's an important concept to understand. A medical professional can't fully understand or appreciate the 12-lead EKG without first understanding wave patterns and their relationship to the direction of electrical conduction through the heart. Understanding that the less the left ventricle is stimulated, the weaker the contraction is, and this causes decreased systemic profusion and increased risk of ventricular arrhythmia. Finally, identification of a shift in cardiac axis can increase suspicion of possible acute or chronic cardiac issue.

Takeaway Notes from Chapter 4:

- *Prehospital cardiac axis focuses on ventricular conduction. Any change in direction of AV current decreases conduction to the left ventricle, thus weakening its capacity to effectively pump.*

- *Structural changes, such as a MI, can alter the QRS deflection as pathways through damaged tissues slow or become impossible for current to navigate.*

- *Whether the QRS appears above or below the isoelectric line is determined by how close a given positive electrode is to the direction of the impulse leaving the AV node. The more the positive electrode of a lead is to the impulse, the more positive (or upright) the QRS will present on the EKG. The farther, the smaller or more negative the QRS.*

- *For the purposes of EMS, the easiest way to determine axis is to simply look at the frontal leads. If leads I, II, and III are all positive, the axis is normal. If they are all negative, this is a right axis. If they are varied, look at aVR (R for Right) and aVL (L for Left). Whichever is positive is your axis shift. This should be followed by examining the lead opposite for negative deflection.*

- *aVR should be negative, unless an electrode is misplaced or a rightward axis shift is present.*

- *Wide complex in V_1 with a downward deflection and a left axis shift confirms a LBBB.*

- *Transporting a symptomatic patient with a potential new-onset LBBB to an appropriate cardiac facility based on your prehospital findings and clinical judgement is never wrong.*

5

Field Interpretation:
The *Meat and Potatoes* of What You Need to Know

Introduction

Each EMS professional will eventually develops his or her style and approach to 12-lead EKG interpretation, yet a starting point is needed to advance any individual effort. This chapter presents a step-by-step method to interpret the 12-lead EKG through the use of patient scenario examples, as well as the introduction of the LEADS mnemonic. Based on my years of prehospital care, I've developed the LEADS approach and believe it's one of the easiest and methodical approaches to the 12-lead EKG.

Quick Caveat

This text is promoting EKG use, yet there are times when a potential cardiac patient would not benefit from a 12-lead EKG. For example, an advanced life support (ALS) unit is four minutes from the closest emergency room offering acute cardiac care. Paramedics arrive to find a 55-year-old male who has the proverbial crushing, substernal chest pain radiating to both arms. He has a history of an MI last year that felt *"exactly the same."* He's pale, sweaty, tachypneic and hypotensive. This is a load-and-go scenario. The priority for this patient is quick stabilization and a cath lab. Clinical judgment must always supersede tools available for a diagnosis. A field EKG offers little when compared to fast transport to a facility offering definitive intervention. As mentioned earlier, gut instinct and clinical judgment must always surpass any machine diagnostics. Never extend scene times to acquire a diagnostic EKG when the patient is not stable, or the diagnosis is evident based on the patient's presentation.

Pattern of Approach for STEMI Diagnosis in the Field Setting

The best way to read a 12-lead EKG within the field setting is to develop a pattern for examining the printout. This pattern of interpretation should always come after a quick view of lead II to ensure no threatening arrhythmias need be addressed. After lead II has been assessed, the most effective starting point is to look for changes in leads viewing the same region of the heart. For example, if changes are found in a lateral lead, look to the next lateral lead for the same findings to confirm your diagnosis. This is done most efficiently by starting at the top left of the EKG, or Lead I, and working downward, looking first for ST change. The following are examples of EKGs using this pattern of diagnosis.

For the following EKG, began at the top left corner or lateral lead I. Within lead I, ST depression is already noted, requiring confirmation in the next adjoining lateral lead, aVL. Note that there is lateral confirmation of ischemia or reciprocal changes.

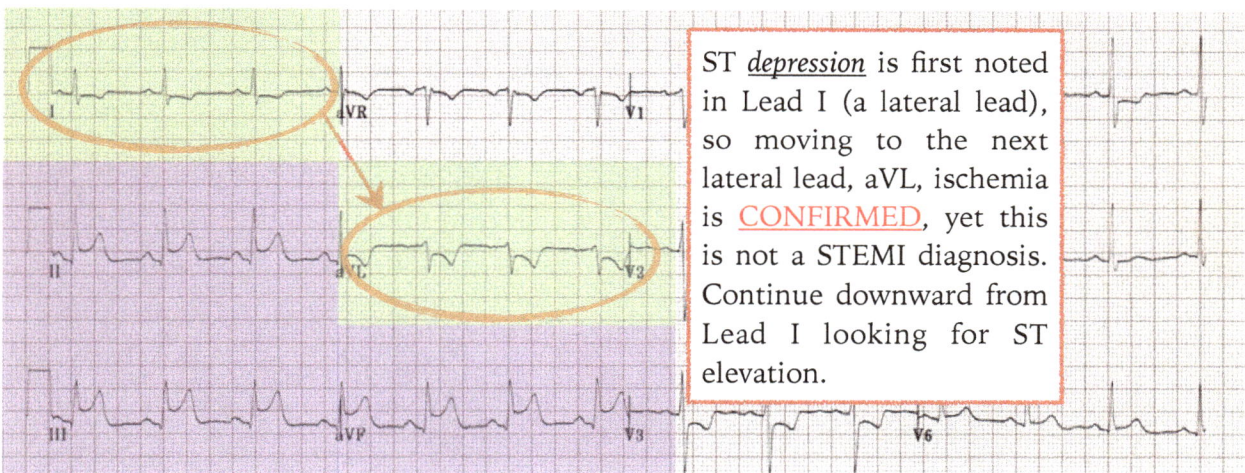

ST *depression* is first noted in Lead I (a lateral lead), so moving to the next lateral lead, aVL, ischemia is CONFIRMED, yet this is not a STEMI diagnosis. Continue downward from Lead I looking for ST elevation.

EKG from litfl.com.

Although it's significant to find ischemic changes in two adjoining leads, it's not diagnostic of a STEMI, as you need ST *elevation* for this diagnosis, so continued examination is needed as these findings may be the result of reciprocal change. It's important to note that in moving from lead I to lead II you're moving from a lateral to an inferior lead. While they're chronological in order, they view different areas of the heart.

Field Interpretation

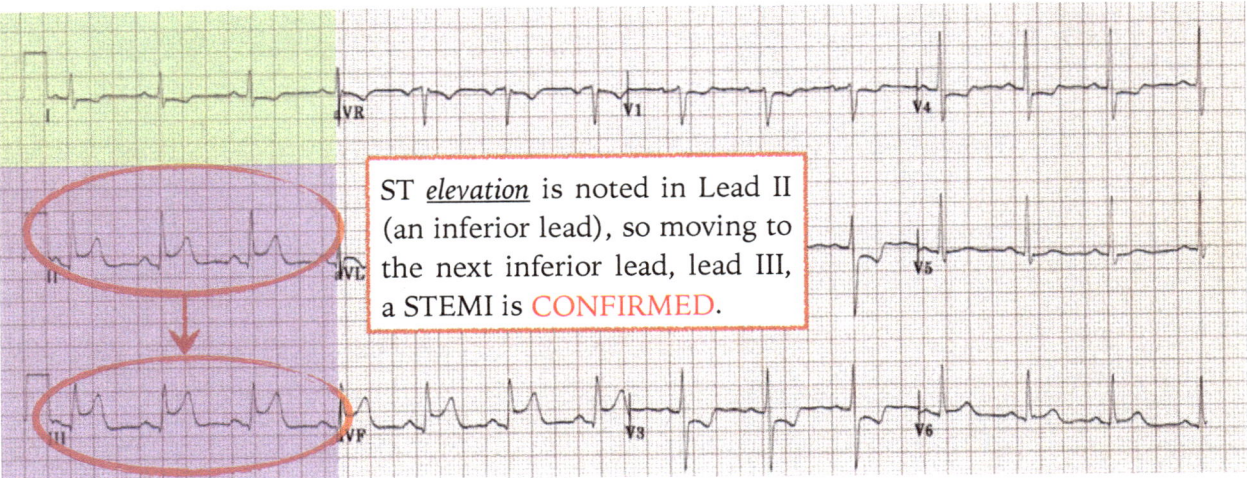

EKG from litfl.com.

Lead II reveals obvious ST elevation. Confirmation then is made by moving to the next inferior lead, lead III, which clearly shows ST elevation as well, thus verifying an inferior STEMI. Essentially, no further interpretation is needed, for the diagnosis is clear in so that a right-sided infarction is considered.

Let's try a not-so-obvious EKG using the same pattern of interpretation, starting with lead I.

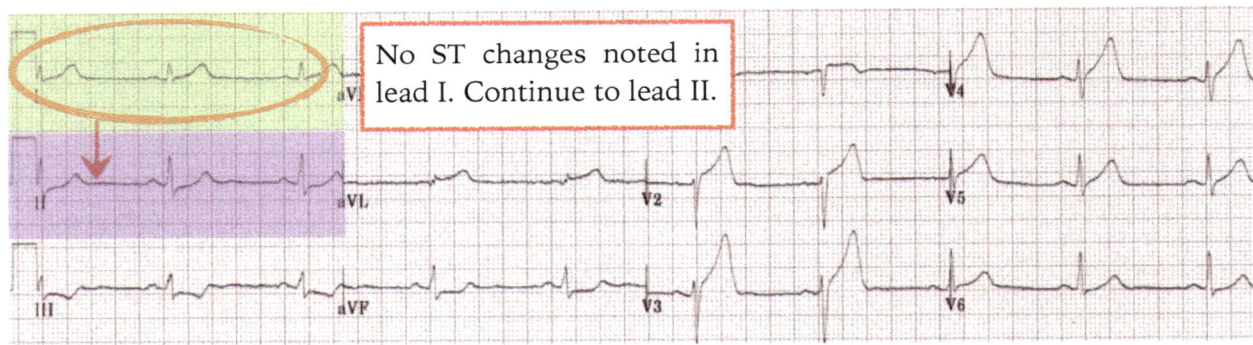

EKG from litfl.com.

Lead I shows no obvious ST changes, therefore we move on (had it shown any ST change, we would move on to the next lateral lead, aVL, to confirm. However, since there are no changes, we move downward to lead II, an inferior lead).

Field Interpretation

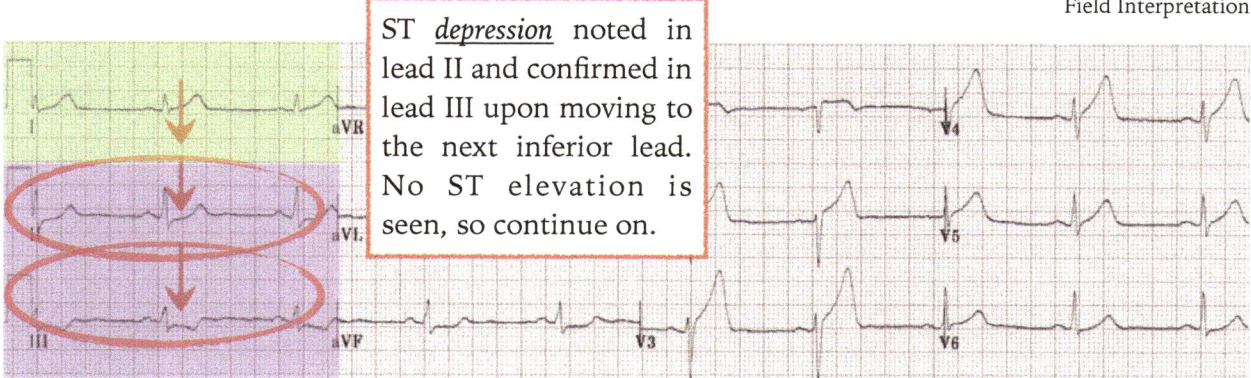

EKG from litfl.com.

Lead II reveals mild ST depression, a sign of ischemia. This is again confirmed by moving to lead III, a consecutive inferior lead, as well as the next step in the interpretation pattern. Lead III confirms ischemic changes, so you know there is cardiac involvement, but is there a STEMI? Is this reciprocal change from a STEMI or is it a NSTEMI? More information is needed to make a diagnosis.

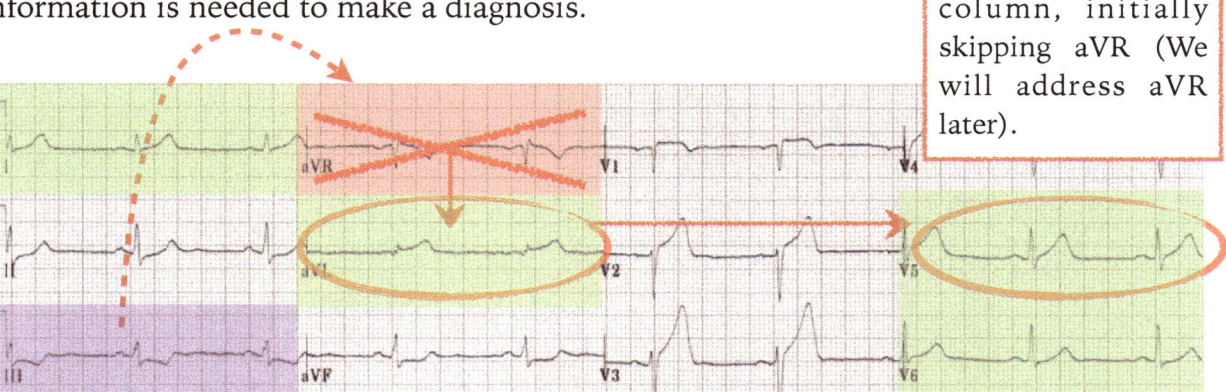

EKG from litfl.com.

From lead III, move to the top of the next column, aVR. Lead aVR offers little information for the initial interpretation (aVR will be addressed further in following sections), so we continue down to aVL. Lead aVL is a lateral lead revealing potential ST

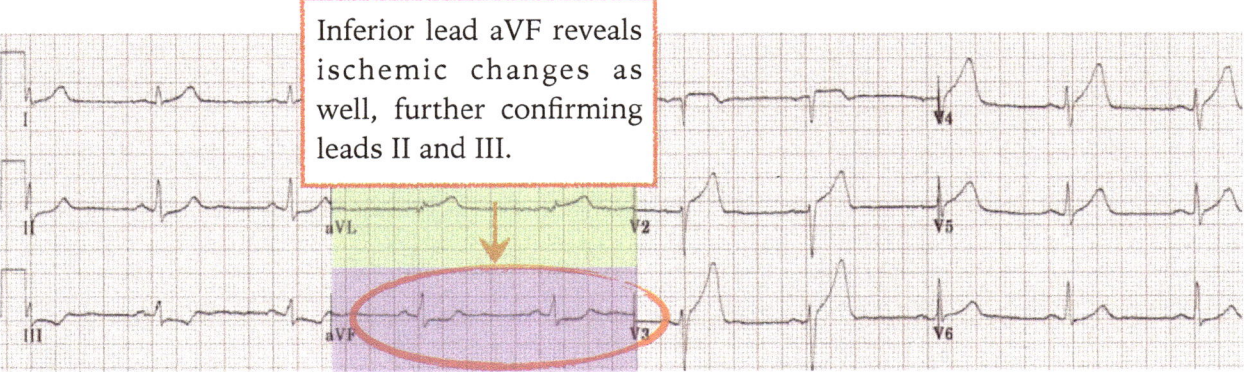

EKG from litfl.com.

39

elevation, prompting a move to the next lateral lead, V$_5$. Lead V$_5$ has a potential hyperacute T wave, indicative of an early infarction, yet no clear ST elevation in V$_5$.

Moving downward from aVL, inferior ischemia is found in aVF (reference next page),

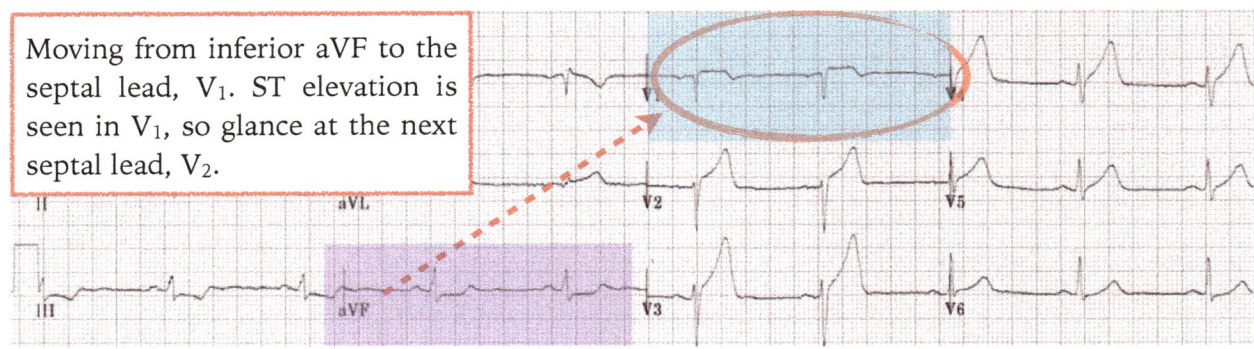

Moving from inferior aVF to the septal lead, V$_1$. ST elevation is seen in V$_1$, so glance at the next septal lead, V$_2$.

EKG from litfl.com.

which is to be expected after inferior leads II and III revealed the same, prompting a move to the top of next column at V$_1$.

Moving from aVF to the top of the next column, we come to lead V$_1$, a septal lead. ST segment elevation is found in V$_1$ and confirmation is made in V$_2$, the next septal lead. ST elevation is also found in V$_3$ and V$_4$, both anterior leads; this confirms an anteroseptal STEMI. Remember, it's common for the septal and anterior leads to bleed from one to the next during an infarction as they are both supplied by the LAD.

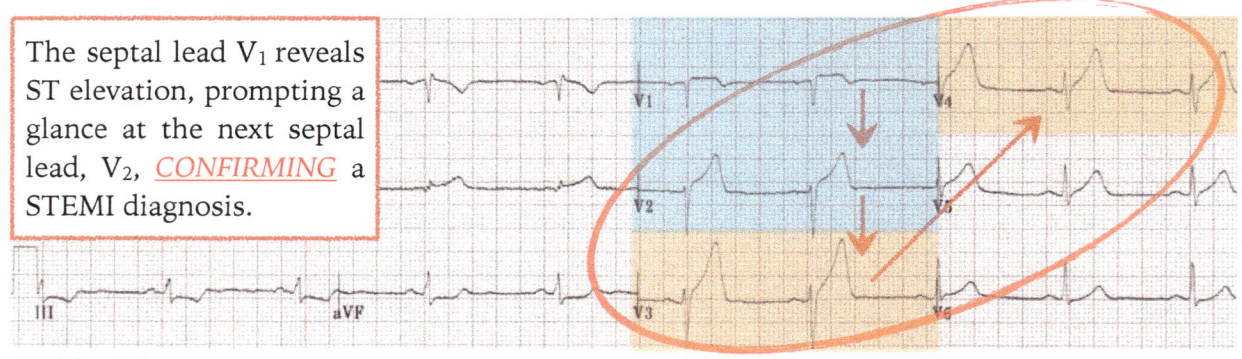

The septal lead V$_1$ reveals ST elevation, prompting a glance at the next septal lead, V$_2$, <u>CONFIRMING</u> a STEMI diagnosis.

EKG from litfl.com.

Formal diagnosis for the above EKG would be an anteroseptal STEMI with reciprocal changes to the inferior leads, resulting from a higher occlusion of the LAD.

Sticking to the same pattern to interpret each and every EKG is paramount to success, and repetitive practice of the method develops a quick means of interpretation. Once the methodology is developed, a whole-picture approach can be learned.

Implementation of the 12-Lead EKG in the Prehospital Environment

In the prehospital setting, the 12-lead EKG is best utilized when both members of the crew understand how to place the electrodes and obtain a readout; either a paramedic or an EMT can attach the EKG. If a second provider obtains the readout, the lead provider can focus on necessary procedures and history taking, allowing for a fluid and efficient scene. Once given the 12-lead EKG is printed, the following page presents a basic approach and pattern of interpretation.

Step 1)   Look at the EKG   *Do all of the leads have clear, discernible rhythms? Is there too much artifact? If unclear, repeat the EKG, if the patient is stable. (If clear, move to Step 2).*

Step 2)   Look at Lead II   *What is the underlying rhythm? Is it lethal (VT, unstable SVT, etc.)? If yes, treat and transport. (If non-lethal, move to Step 3).*

Step 3)   Look for ST changes   *STEMI or NSTEMI? If ST change is found, is it seen in two adjoining leads? If so, transport quickly to a cardiac center. (If not, move to Step 4).*

Step 4)   Look at the axis   *Normal? Shifted left? Look at V_1. Does this confirm a LBBB diagnosis? Is a new-onset LBBB suspected? If so, consult with your receiving hospital or transport to the nearest cardiac center. (If not, move to Step 5).*

Step 5)   Look at the patient's symptoms   *Probable Non-STEMI? Consider differentials (Aortic aneurysm/dissection, PE, pneumothorax, etc.), and transport accordingly.*

This five-step pattern provides a primary means of interpretation, so remember, only look for immediate threats. Subtle or superfluous findings, such as ventricular strains, hemiblocks, or hypertrophy (not discussed in this textbook), are not pertinent for the field setting. The time needed to review the EKG in the prehospital setting should be brief and focused; don't overthink, as this leads to tunnel vision and less time treating the patient. Think your way through your diagnostic EKG pattern.

For those who benefit from acronyms, I have come up with the *"LEADS"* acronym. We'll utilize this approach further in Chapter 6.

L	*Lead II?*	*What's the underlying rhythm?*
		Does it require treatment?
		Yes, stop and treat accordingly; no, continue.
E	*EKG Changes?*	*ST depression/elevation/Q waves?*
		If yes, stop and transport accordingly;
		If no, continue.
A	*Axis?*	*Normal, left, or right?*
		Likely new onset LBBB?
		If yes, consider and continue.
D	*Differentials?*	*Are there any signs or symptoms concerning for other potential life-threatening differentials (thoracic or abdominal aneurysm, dissection, pneumothorax vs. other)?*
		Yes, stop and treat accordingly; no, continue.
S	*Stability?*	*Is there an immediate concern for impending arrest or chance of sudden deterioration?*
		Yes, stop and treat accordingly; no, transport accordingly.

For those who prefer an algorithmic approach to learning, the following page offers a visual approach to interpretation (*figure 5.1*). Any approach is appropriate, as long as there's no deviation from it.

Once the QRS morphologies, patterns, and associations on the EKG are understood, diagnosis is relatively straightforward, so practice and repeat. Is lead II a lethal rhythm? If not, are there ST changes? Are those ST changes in adjoining leads? Do they reveal ST depression (NSTEMI) or ST elevation (STEMI)? Done. Keeping it simple clears the thought process. Too many prehospital providers overthink things that could be very simple.

As shown, there are several ways to approach this information, yet the key is to stay focused, look for visible signs, and go with your gut. Keep it simple. If the patient is hemodynamically stable, there's time to obtain an EKG. If that EKG is clean but the patient looks awful, load-and-go. Whether it's cardiac or not, the patient isn't stable.

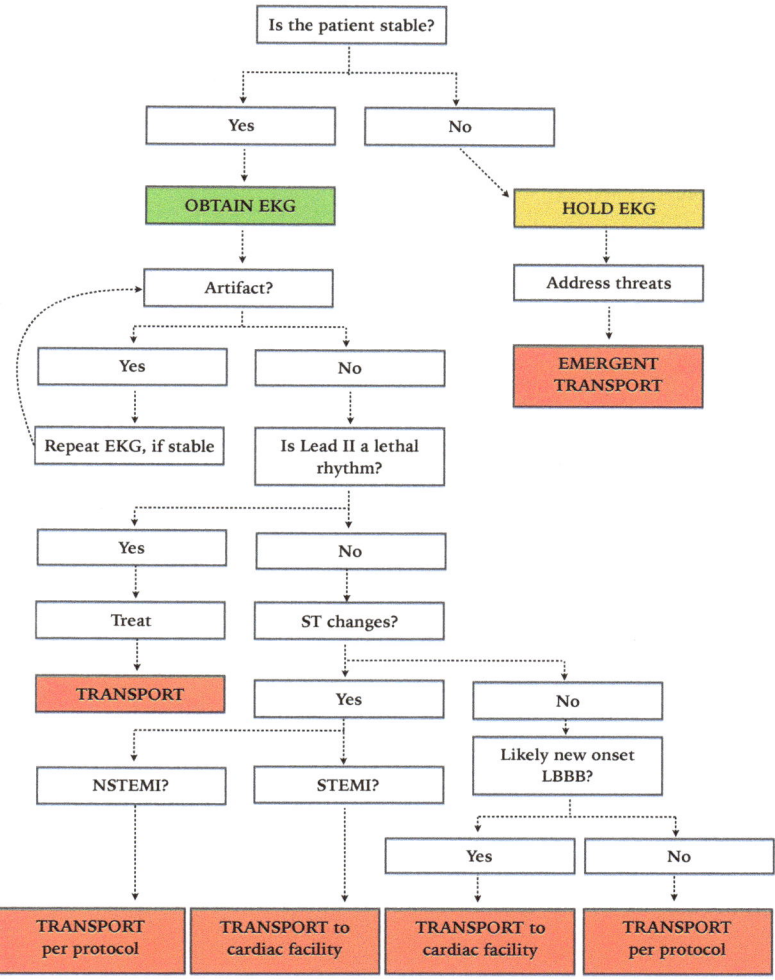

Figure 5.1: *Algorithmic Approach to 12-Lead Interpretation in the Prehospital Setting.*

It may be imperative to forgo the EKG in order to stabilize the patient and transport to the nearest, appropriate facility. If time allows, obtain an EKG only after everything else is addressed (i.e., airway, breathing, blood pressure, pulse, differentials). Implement one method into your practice and stick with it for every patient until it becomes an effortless pattern to follow. Let's practice.

Scenario 1:

(Use the provided reference on the back of the book for the following scenarios)

You arrive to find a 42-year-old, obese male sitting at a kitchen table, complaining of chest *"tightness"* for one hour after eating. He's taken four Tums® without relief. He states that the pain is non-radiating and is *"making it difficult to catch my breath."* He has a history of hypertension, hyperlipidemia, and smokes one pack of cigarettes daily. He takes three medications that he cannot remember.

He denies recent illness, fever, chills, cough, nausea, vomiting, abdominal pain, back or flank pain, dizziness, syncope, and headache. These are *pertinent negatives*, intended to narrow the diagnosis down to its most likely cause.

His vital signs are: blood pressure 170/90; pulse 90; respirations 24; saturations are 94%.

He's alert and oriented, pink and dry, and his lungs are clear. No palpable masses are noted to his abdomen, and he has equal radial and pedal pulses. There's mild, 2+, non-pitting edema noted to both ankles.

Your partner places the patient on oxygen and the 3-lead monitor as you look for an IV site. You are given the strip of the 3-lead printout while your partner prepares the 12-lead EKG for placement.

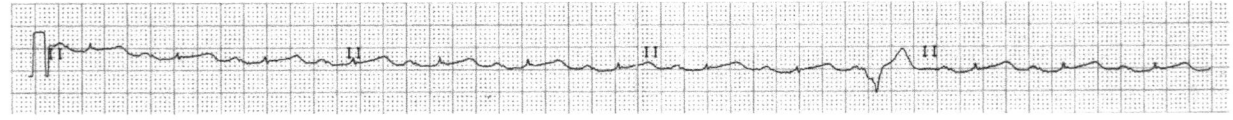

EKG from litfl.com.

Is this rhythm lethal? No. The rate is stable and a PVC is noted. There are no concerns that need be addressed now.

Is this patient stable enough for a 12-lead EKG in the field? Yes. He has no immediate threats. He's conscious and breathing adequately. His heart and blood pressure are stable for the moment.

Field Interpretation

A intravenous catheter (IV) is secured and 324 milligrams of aspirin is administered orally as your partner hands you the 12-lead EKG printout.

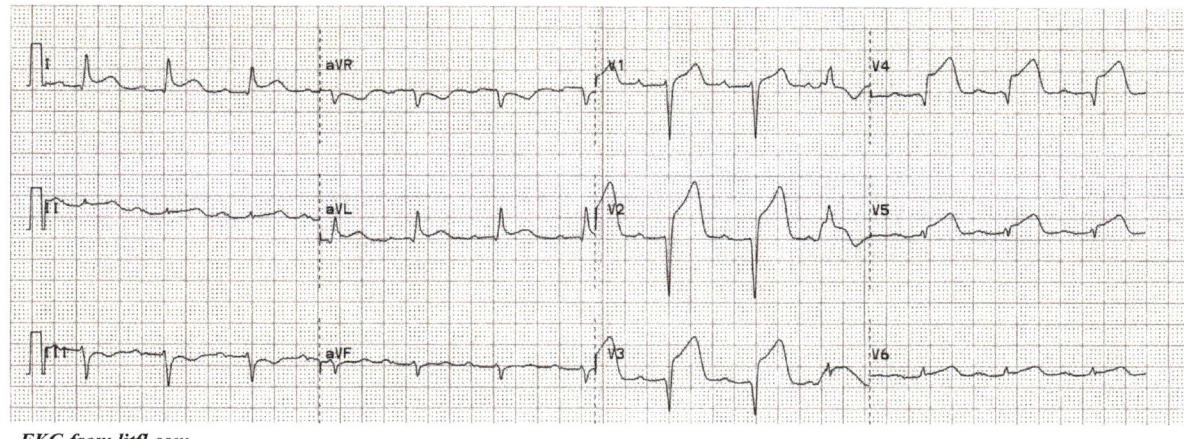

EKG from litfl.com.

Is this EKG concerning? YES.

The EKG shows a clear **anteroseptal STEMI with lateral involvement** (*figure 5.2*). There's no ST elevation in aVR, so a LMCA is ruled out; There's no overt reciprocal change, yet this is an obvious STEMI with concern for a high LAD. Nitroglycerin is appropriate for this patient as his blood pressure is stable and there are no signs of an inferior infarct. Time to move! There's no need to look at the axis because the diagnosis is quite clear.

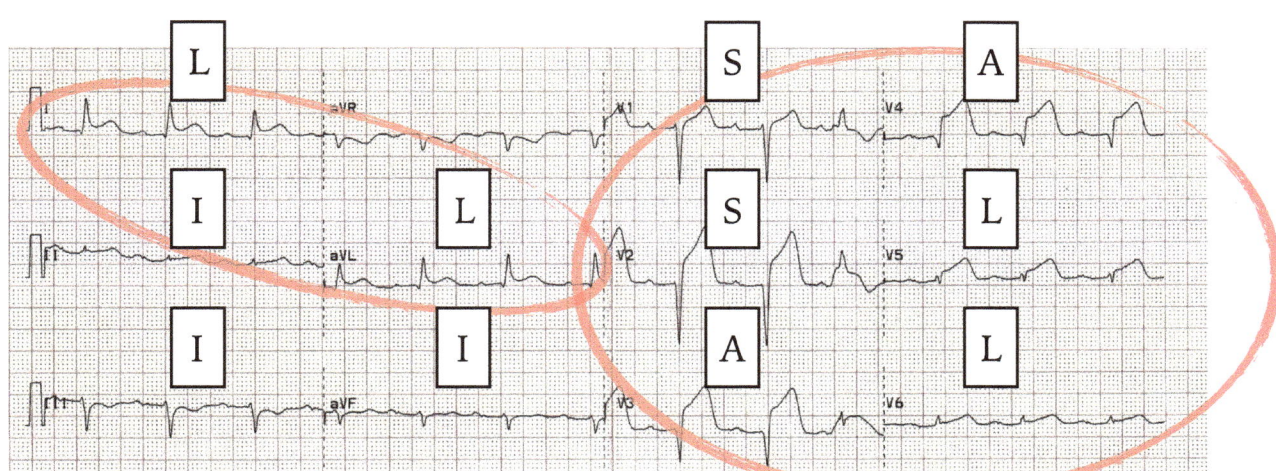

Figure 5.2: Anteroseptal STEMI with Lateral Involvement using the "LII, LI, SSAALL" Method. EKG from litfl.com.

Scenario 2:

You arrive to find an 80-year-old female complaining of weakness, nausea, and vomiting for one day. She denies fever, chills, shortness of breath, abdominal pain, back pain, dizziness, and syncope. She states that she awoke in the night with these symptoms, and no one else in the home has been ill. She has an extensive history including insulin-dependent diabetes, hypertension, peripheral vascular disease, congestive heart failure, and two cardiac stents. She takes Spironolactone, Lisinopril, Levemir, Novolog, and a daily aspirin.

Her vital signs are: blood pressure 104/78; Pulse of 78; respirations are 20; saturations are 97%.

She's alert and oriented, pink, and warm. Her lung sounds are diminished without rales, rhonchi, or wheeze. No abdominal tenderness or pulsating masses. She has equal pulses. No obvious peripheral edema noted.

You start an IV and administer 4 milligrams of Ondansetron as your partner places the patient on four LPM of oxygen via nasal cannula and places the 3-lead EKG.

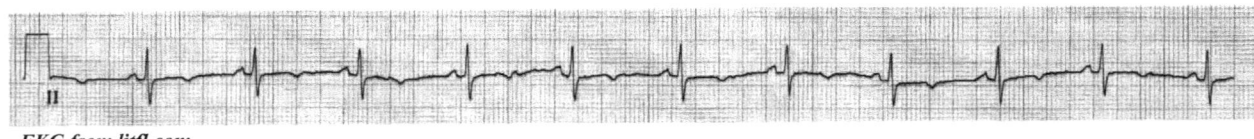

EKG from litfl.com.

Is this rhythm lethal? No. However, there is T-wave inversion to note.

Is this patient stable enough for a 12-lead in the field? Yes.

Your partner readies the 12-lead EKG. After acquiring a printout, she hands the readout to you (see next page).

Field Interpretation

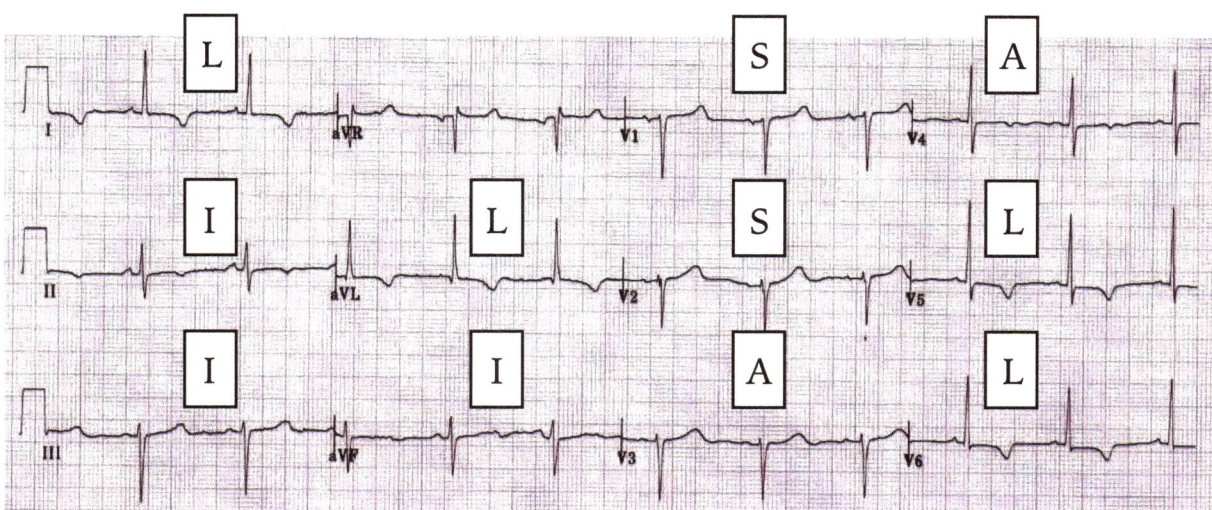

EKG from litfl.com.

Is this EKG concerning? Yes.

Recall in Chapter 2 when we discussed the progression of an MI and STEMI versus NSTEMI. A STEMI is represented by *ST elevation* whereas a NSTEMI is ST change *other than* ST elevation, often representing ischemia, or a lack of oxygen to a given region. ST depression or T-wave inversion represent ischemic changes and meets NSTEMI criteria when it's found in two adjoining leads. Looking again at the EKG (*figure 5.3*), what are the changes and where are they located? This EKG reveals *T-wave inversion within the lateral leads* (I, aVL, V_5, V_6). While T-wave inversion is also found in lead II, there are no similar findings within the other inferior leads, thus lacking criteria for inferior involvement.

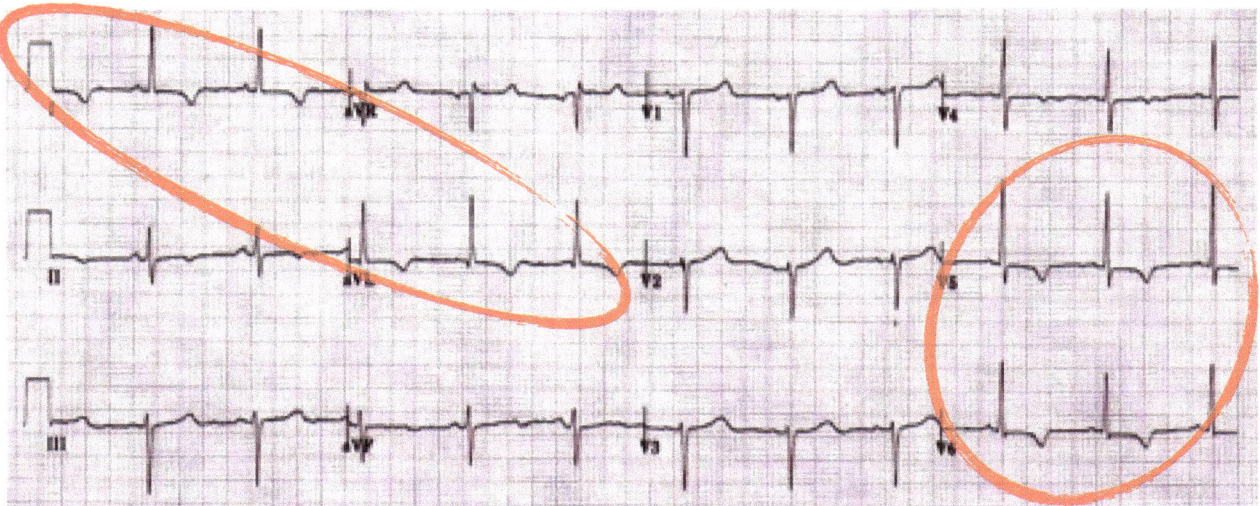

Figure 5.3: *Lateral T Wave Inversion in Leads I, aVL, V_{5-6}. EKG from litfl.com.*

What is your treatment?

Aspirin and nitroglycerin are appropriate for this patient as her blood pressure is stable and there's no sign of an inferior infarct. Since this is classified as a NSTEMI, transportation to the closest facility is appropriate; however, don't be surprised if they divert you to a cardiac center. If you complete serial EKGs after your nitroglycerin dosing, it's possible to see the signs of ischemia diminish or clear, or the patient develop ST segment elevation.

Scenario 3:

You arrive to find a 52-year-old male complaining of substernal chest pain for 30 minutes. The onset was sudden and radiates to both arms, and his symptoms are accompanied by shortness of breath. He cannot tell you his past medical history, but his wife hands you his medications, which include Metformin, Diltiazem, Glipizide, nitroglycerin, ipratropium bromide/albuterol sulfate, Lorsartan, and aspirin.

He's not able to provide pertinent negatives due to distress.

He's alert, pale, and sweaty. There are rales throughout the his lower lung fields. He has no abdominal pain or obvious pulsating mass. His pulses are equal and strong. 1+ pitting edema is noted to his feet and ankles.

His vital signs are 214/P on the right arm and 210/P on the left; pulse 90, irregular; respirations of 30; and his oxygen saturations are 92%.

Your partner places the patient on high flow oxygen and hands you the 3-lead EKG.

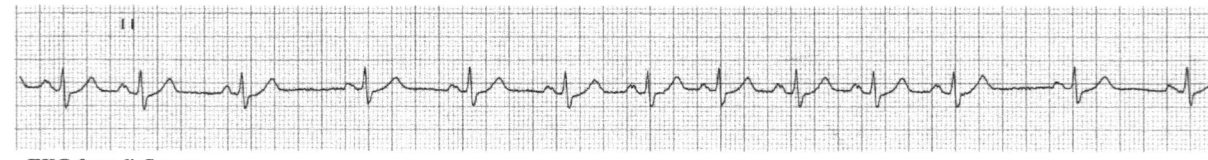

EKG from litfl.com.

Is this rhythm concerning? No.

Is this patient stable enough for time to obtain a 12-lead EKG? No.

This is a load-and-go patient. This man is a clearly distressed patient who's at risk for arrest based on their initial presentation, so oxygen, intravenous access, aspirin (if appropriate), and emergent transport are priorities before any 12-lead is obtained. Unstable cardiac patients benefit most from quick specialty intervention, not your EKG, so head for the cardiac center. Gut instinct should always outshine anything a machine can offer.

What are three differentials to consider other than a myocardial infarction with the given scenario?

1. Thoracic or abdominal aneurysm/dissection
2. Pulmonary embolism
3. Pneumothorax

A well-respected emergency room physician once told me anything that comes on fast and strong is probably a bad thing (i.e. thoracic aneurysm, cerebral hemorrhage, etc.), and bad things often don't get better with initial diagnostics or treatments (i.e., EKG, medications, etc.).

Scenario 3 also stresses the importance of a basic knowledge of the common prescribed home medications as they're a tool to acquire a patient's history when either the patient is unable to give it or they don't know it. I can't tell you how many times a look in the patient's purse (with permission) or a browse through their bathroom cabinet told me the story that I needed to know. Here's a listing of this patient's medications and their common use:

1. Metformin: Diabetes
2. Diltiazem: Atrial fibrillation/hypertension
3. Glipizide: Diabetes
4. Nitroglycerin: Angina
5. Ipratropium bromide/albuterol sulfate: COPD/Asthma
6. Lorsartan: Blood pressure
7. Aspirin: Anti-platelet

It is important to note that that all of these medications are given to patients with conditions that increase the likelihood of cardiovascular disease and an acute coronary event such as an MI.

Scenario 4:

You arrive on scene to find a 60-year-old male complaining of nausea, vomiting and chest pressure for four hours, and he thinks he has *"the flu."*. He has no significant history except a cholecystectomy in 2012. He takes multi-vitamins and aspirin daily, *"Because my wife tells me to."*

When you ask about pertinent negatives, he denies fevers, chills, shortness of breath, abdominal pain, diarrhea, constipation, back pain, headache, dizziness, syncope or increased pain with movement or palpation.

Quick review: *Why would you ask about the above pertinent negatives?*
1. Fever/chills: Possible infectious pathology
2. Shortness of breath: Pneumothorax, CHF, bronchospasm, pneumonia, embolism
3. Abdominal pain: AAA, cardiac, gastrointestinal
4. Diarrhea/constipation: Infectious, obstructive vs other
5. Back pain: Aneurysm, renal, musculoskeletal
6. Headache: Aneurysm, TIA, CVA
7. Dizziness/syncope: Possible neurological pathology, cardiac, embolism
8. Provocative pain: Musculoskeletal vs other

Patients with lower risk factors require consideration of differentials. So many field paramedics hear *"chest pain"* and go straight to aspirin and nitroglycerin. Think about your differentials, ask your pertinent negatives.

Your patient's vital signs are: blood pressure 170/80; pulse 88; respirations 14; oxygen saturations of 98%.

He's alert and oriented; pale, yet warm and dry.

Quick review: *Why are these areas important for the physical exam?*
1. Skin signs: Color, temperature, moisture clue you into the patients stability. Diaphoresis is never a good sign.
2. Lungs: tight, wheezing: asthma, COPD, cardiac; rhonchi: infectious, COPD; rales: pneumonia, CHF; absent or asymmetry: pneumothorax.
3. Abdomen: mass, pulsations: AAA, dissection.
4. Pulses: unequal: AAA, dissection; weak: shock; irregular: arrhythmia.
5. Peripheral edema: heart failure, vascular obstruction, pulmonary embolism.

Your cardiac exam reveals an irregular rate, though he has strong, equal pulses. His lungs are clear and abdomen soft, non-tender, and without mass or pulsations. There's no peripheral edema to note.

Your partner places the patient on four liters via nasal cannula and attaches the 3-lead monitor as you ready your IV supplies.

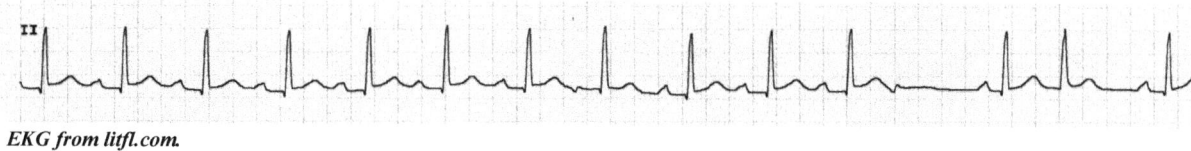

EKG from litfl.com.

Is this rhythm lethal? No.

Is there anything to note? Yes.

It appears that there may be some ST elevation. Remember lead II views the inferior portion of the heart supplied by the right coronary artery.

Do you have time to attach the 12-lead monitor for a reading? Yes. The patient is stable.

Your partner attaches the 12-lead electrodes as you acquire IV access and administer four milligrams of Ondansetron. Here's your 12-lead printout:

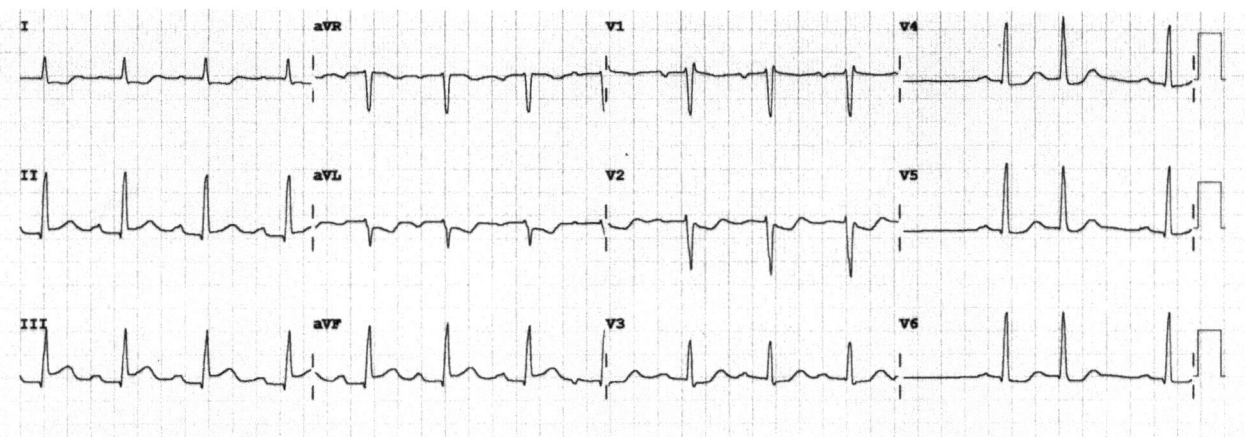

EKG from litfl.com.

Is this 12-lead concerning? Yes.

This patient is having an *inferior STEMI*, as shown in leads II, III, aVF with mild reciprocal change in the anteroseptal (consider posterior involvement) and lateral leads. Recognizing this pattern, you initiate rapid transport to the cardiac center. After administering 324 milligrams of aspirin by mouth and 0.4 milligrams of nitroglycerin sublingually, the patient begins to feel short of breath and lightheaded. You check his radial pulse, and can't find one. He's very pale in appearance compared to when you arrived, yet remains alert. His heart rate is now 110. You quickly place him in Trendelenburg, open his normal saline drip wide open, and recheck his blood pressure: 78/40.

What happened?

Recall our discussion of inferior infarctions in Chapter 3. It's important to consider the possibility of a right ventricular infarct in these patients, as they're sensitive to preload changes.

After administering 500 milliliters of normal saline, the patient's color improves as does his lightheadedness. You move the V₄ electrode to the exact same position on the right breast and print another EKG labeling V₄ as "V₄R." You note the ST elevation in V₄R, confirming a right-ventricular or right-sided infarction (*figure 5.4*). His blood pressure is now 112/88. Further nitroglycerin doses should be withheld.

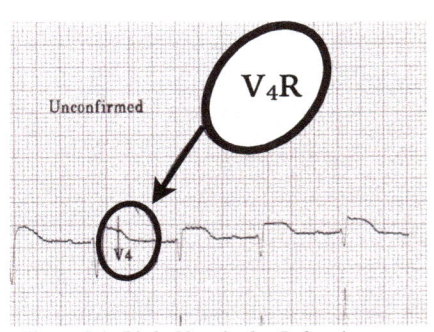

Figure 5.4: *Right Ventricular Infarction as Represented by V₄R. EKG from litfl.com.*

Scenario 5:

You arrive to find a 39-year-old man complaining of shortness of breath and chest *"tightness,"* which began 10 minutes ago while he was running a marathon. He tells you that he just felt *"winded"* during the race before the chest discomfort started and he has never felt like this before. He has no cardiac or other medical history. He takes no medications.

He denies fevers, chills, cough, abdominal pain, back pain, headache, dizziness, syncope or increased pain with movement or palpation.

His vital signs are: blood pressure 148/70; pulse 88; respirations 26; oxygen saturations of 96%.

He's alert and oriented, warm and dry. He has a regular heart rate. His lungs are clear and abdomen soft, non-tender, without mass or pulsations. He has strong, equal pulses. There's no peripheral edema to note.

The patient is placed on a nasal cannula and 3-lead monitor.

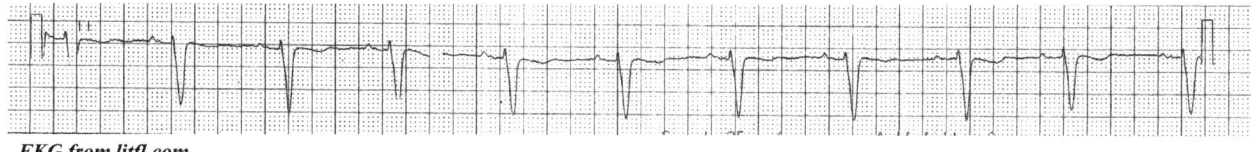

EKG from litfl.com.

Is this rhythm lethal? No. However, it is concerning due to the increased QRS width.

This patient, who told you that he has *"no cardiac history,"* has a widened QRS complex >1.2 millimeters suggesting a bundle branch block. A bundle branch block makes it difficult to interpret an infarct without a prior comparison EKG. Despite this, an EKG needs to be obtained, if only to confirm that the patient indeed has a LBBB.

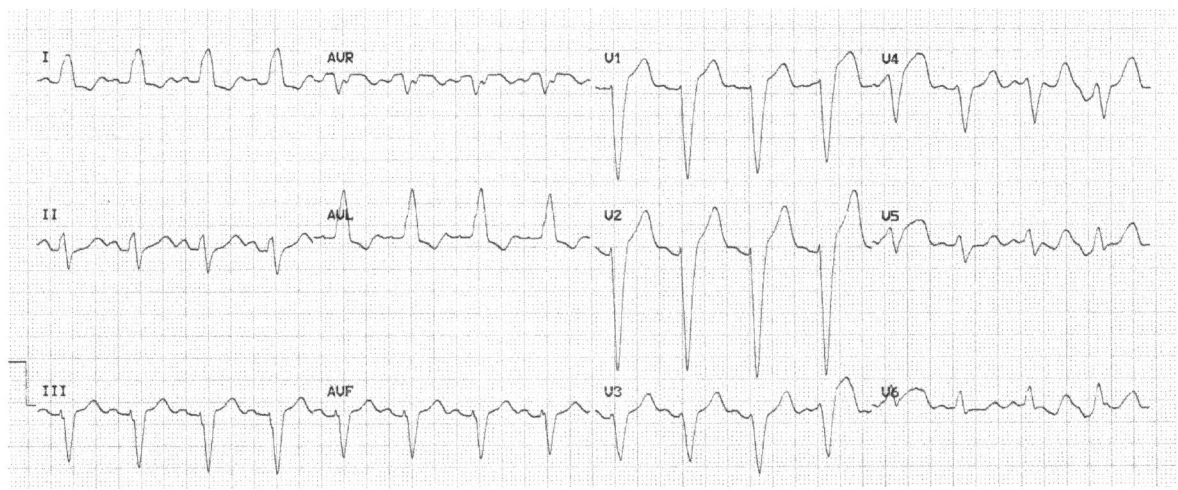

EKG from litfl.com.

Is this 12-lead concerning? *Yes*

This patient *does* have a LBBB, which is highly concerning of a cardiac cause for his symptoms. A healthy patient, *without* cardiac history, *should not* have a LBBB. While not considered STEMI criteria, one should remain suspicious of the patient's complaints and EKG findings. Transport decision-making should be made using sound clinical judgment, and consultation with your base hospital is beneficial for determining transport when your patient has a new-onset LBBB. These patients require a high level of clinical acumen for they are at risk for an underlying anteroseptal infarction.

This chapter discussed several approaches to applying the 12-lead EKG to prehospital practice. Developing a repetitive, simple method is imperative, and application of this method to every 12-lead EKG interpretation reduces the chance of error. Over time, this method will become second nature and findings will quickly stand out, further enhancing confidence and field judgment. Only through continuous practice can proficiency be obtained.

Takeaway Notes for Chapter 5:

- *While chest pain is the most common complaint requiring a 12-lead EKG, it's not the only complaint that it's useful for.*

- *There are significant differences in complaints between men and women during an acute MI, and additional differences in the elderly. Females may present with atypical symptoms of fatigue, nausea, throat, shoulder, and back pain.*

- *When interpreting an EKG, remember to look for similarities in leads that represent the same area of the heart (e.g. inferior II and III, lateral V_5 and V_6, etc.).*

- *Never allow a 12-lead EKG to supplant gut instinct born of strong clinical judgment. These skills will always trump any machine at your disposal. Never extend scene times to acquire a diagnostic EKG when the patient isn't stable, or the diagnosis is clear due to the patient's presentation.*

- *Once you understand the morphologies, patterns, and associations on the EKG, diagnosis is fairly straightforward.*

- *Keeping things simple clears your mind of superfluous information that fogs a focused, critical thinking process. Too many prehospital providers overthink things that could be left very simple.*

- *Develop one method of interpretation and never deviate from that approach. Your singular approach is an efficient means to develop proficiency.*

6

The LEADS Approach to Prehospital 12-Lead EKG Interpretation

This chapter is pure practice. A total of 10 EKGs are presented using the LEADS pattern for interpretation. Each EKG has an attached scenario to follow. As you practice, it's essential that the same pattern is used to analyze every EKG. A reliable guide increases efficiency and decreases the frequency of error. Additionally, a singular approach allows for a broader understanding of more subtle concerns, such as a LMCA or posterior infarction. I encourage you to use the attached 12-lead EKG reference found on the back of the book when interpreting the following scenarios.

Good luck!

LEADS ALGORITHM
WITH PATIENT PRESENTATIONS

The LEADS Pattern of Interpretation

L *Lead II?*

  - Does lead II reveal a lethal rhythm that requires immediate intervention?

E *EKG Changes?*

  - Any evidence of a STEMI or NSTEMI in two leads viewing the same region of the heart?

A *Axis Change?*

  - Any evidence of an axis shift giving rise to a potential left bundle branch block (LBBB)?

D *Differentials?*

  - Any signs or symptoms concerning for life threatening differentials?

S *Stability?*

  - Any signs or symptoms showing concern for an impending arrest or deterioration?

EKG #1

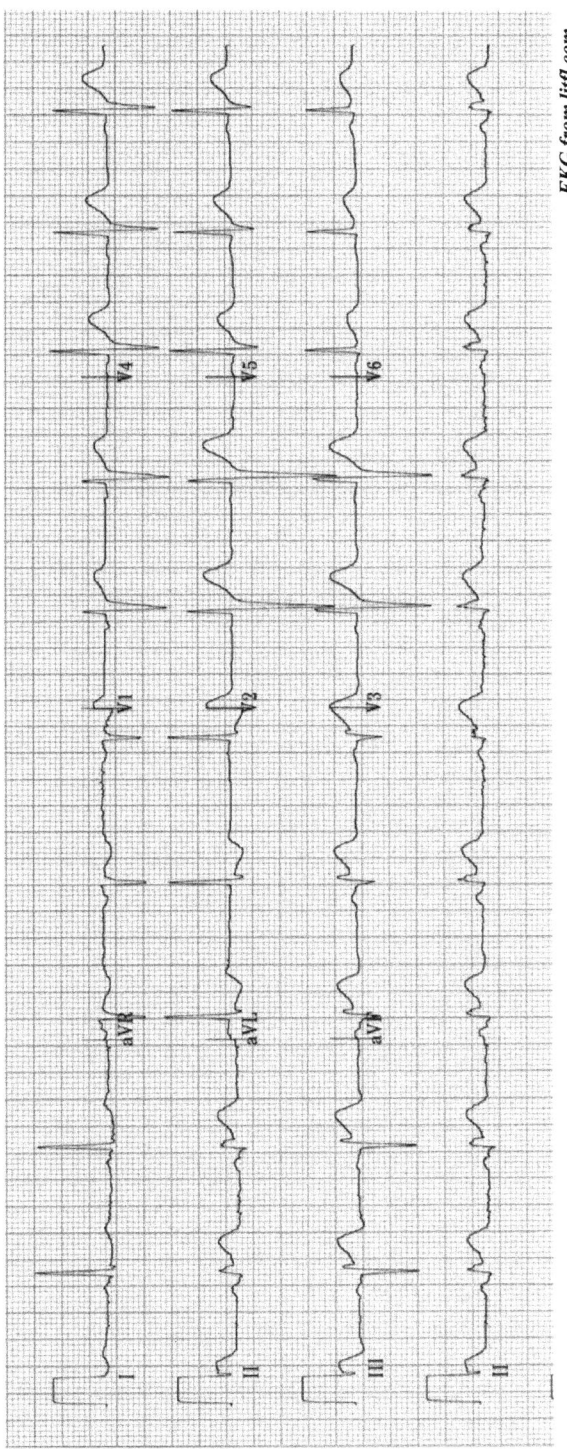

EKG from litfl.com

You arrive on scene to find a 55-year-old male complaining of *"chest pressure"* for three hours. He states the pressure came on after mowing the lawn. He attempted to rest, yet it hasn't resolved. His only history includes diet-controlled high cholesterol. Vitals signs are: blood pressure 130/90; heart rate 72 and regular; respirations are 20 with saturations of 96%. He's alert and oriented. His skin is pink, warm, and moist. His lungs are clear and abdomen benign. No edema is noted and pulses are equal throughout your exam.

L   *Lead II?*   _____

E   *EKG Changes?*   _____

A   *Axis Change?*   _____

D   *Differentials?*   _____

S   *Stability?*   _____

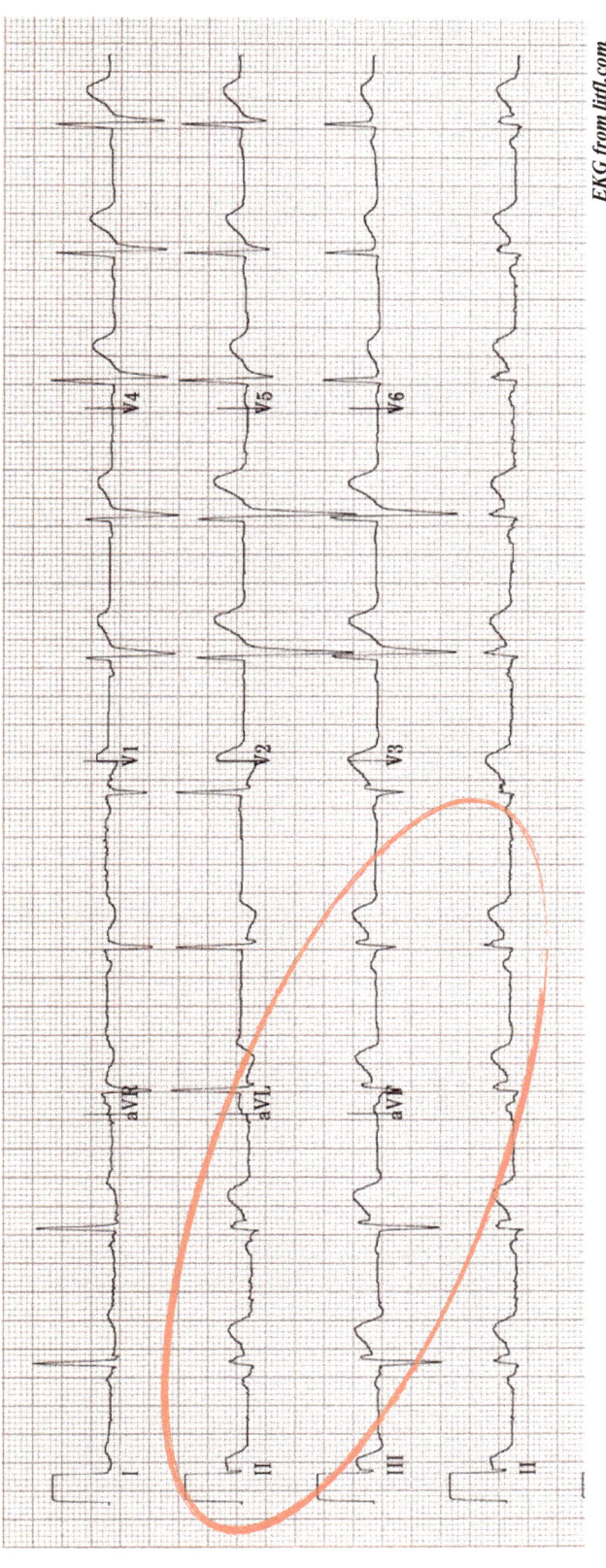

L *Lead II?* SINUS RHYTHM WITH OBVIOUS ST SEGMENT ELEVATION.

E *EKG Changes?* CLEAR INFERIOR STEMI.

A *Axis Change?* LEFT AXIS DEVIATION; HOWEVER, NO EVIDENCE OF LBBB.

D *Differentials?* CONSIDER RIGHT VENTRICULAR INFARCTION.

S *Stability?* CURRENTLY STABLE, YET RAPID TRANSPORT IS NEEDED.

EKG #2

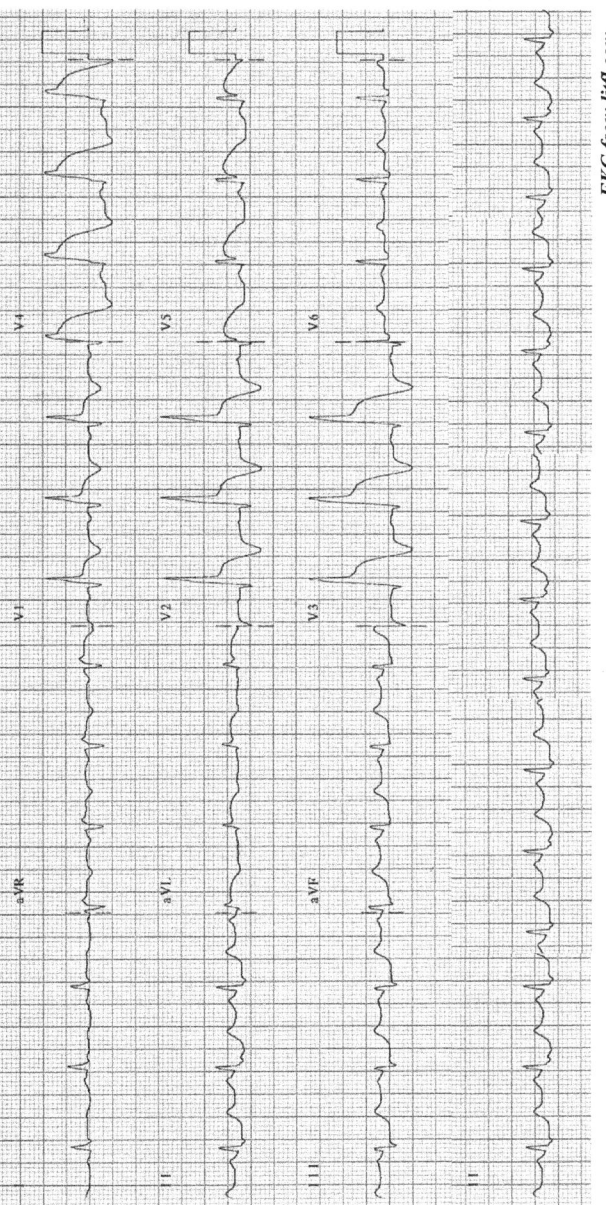

EKG from litfl.com

You arrive on scene to find a 52-year-old, obese male sitting outside a diner, complaining of substernal chest *"pressure"* for 20 minutes. He states that he finished his hamburger and stepped out for a cigarette when the pressure gradually came on. When asked about his history, he states *"I'm healthy,"* and that he doesn't take any medications. His vital signs are: blood pressure of 162/80; heart rate of 90, regular; respirations of 30; and saturations of 96%. He's pale, warm, yet sweaty; his lungs are diminished bilaterally; his abdomen is without pulsating mass; no overt edema is noted and his pulses are equal.

L   *Lead II?* _____

E   *EKG Changes?* _____

A   *Axis Change?* _____

D   *Differentials?* _____

S   *Stability?* _____

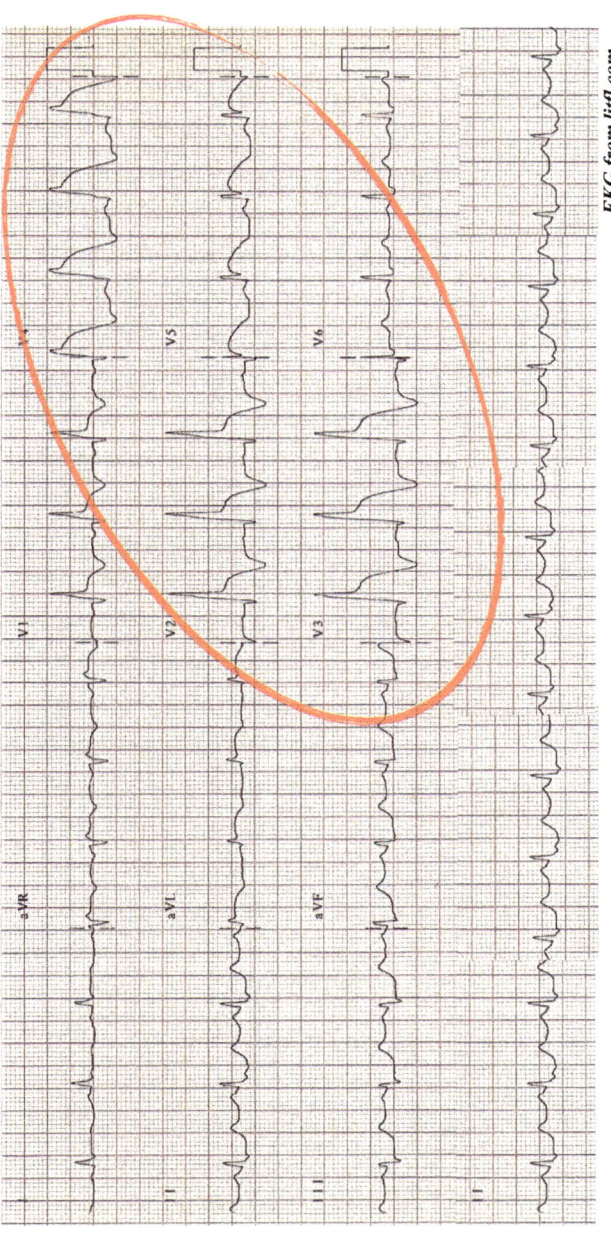

EKG from litfl.com

L	*Lead II?*	SINUS RHYTHM WITH ST DEPRESSION.
E	*EKG Changes?*	ST ELEVATION NOTED TO THE SEPTAL, ANTERIOR, AND V_5 WITH RECIPROCAL CHANGES INFERIORLY.
A	*Axis Change?*	NO.
D	*Differentials?*	NONE.
S	*Stability?*	HIGH CONCERN FOR IMPENDING ARREST.

EKG #3

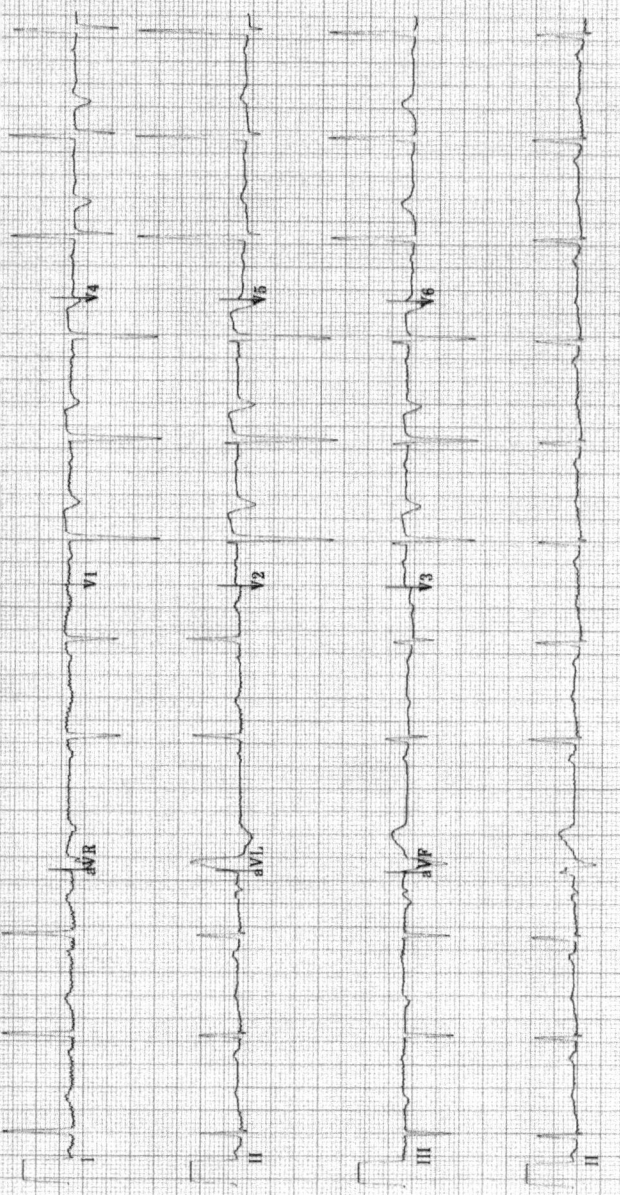

EKG from litfl.com

You arrive on scene to find a 70-year-old female sitting at a card table, complaining of sudden onset throat and bilateral shoulder pain. She states she was playing bridge when the symptoms came on rapidly and now she's having difficulty breathing. She states she may have *"pulled something decorating"* an hour before. She takes *"several blood pressure medications,"* including a *"water pill"* and potassium. Her vital signs reveal a blood pressure 202/102; heart rate of 72; respirations of 32 and labored; and saturations of 92%. She's pale, warm, and dry; her lungs are clear bilaterally; her abdomen is without pulsating mass; her pulses are equal and no peripheral edema. noted.

L   *Lead II?*   _____

E   *EKG Changes?*   _____

A   *Axis Change?*   _____

D   *Differentials?*   _____

S   *Stability?*   _____

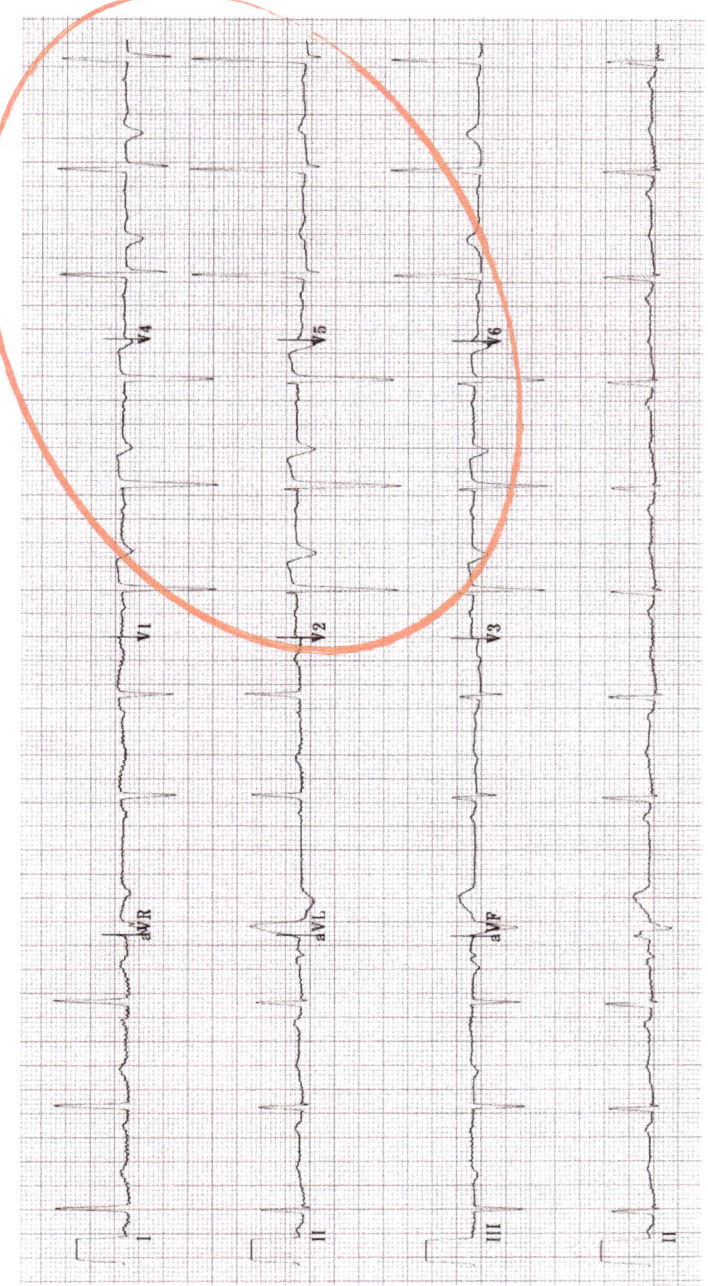

EKG from litfl.com

L	*Lead II?*	SINUS RHYTHM WITH PVC.
E	*EKG Changes?*	T-WAVE CHANGES TO THE SEPTAL AND ANTERIOR LEADS.
A	*Axis Change?*	LEFT AXIS WITH NO EVIDENCE OF LBBB.
D	*Differentials?*	NSTEMI VS ANEURSYM VS PULMONARY EMBOLISM VS EARLY POSTERIOR INFARCTION.***
S	*Stability?*	HIGH CONCERN FOR IMPENDING DETERIORATION.

***While not addressed in this text, this T-wave pattern is suggestive of Wellen's Syndrome, representative of an underlying stenosis of the proximal LAD.

EKG #4

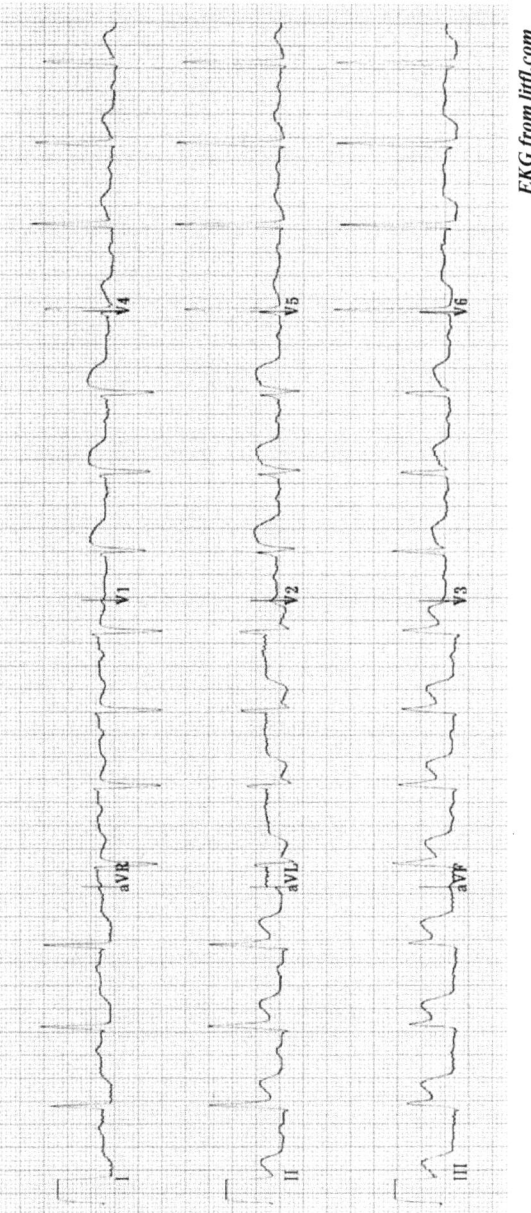

EKG from lifl.com

You arrive on scene to find a 42-year-old male leaning against a work bench in his garage, complaining of gradual onset chest and left arm pain for six hours. He has a history of insulin-dependent diabetes, angina, COPD, and psoriasis. He wasn't able to find his nitroglycerin tablets because he *"hasn't had to take them in a long time."* His vital signs are blood pressure 138/72; heart rate of 82; respirations of 20 and saturations of 99%. He's pink, warm, and dry; his lungs are clear bilaterally; his abdomen is without pulsating mass; his pulses are equal with no peripheral edema noted.

L   *Lead II?*   NOT GIVEN

E   *EKG Changes?*   _____

A   *Axis Change?*   _____

D   *Differentials?*   _____

S   *Stability?*   _____

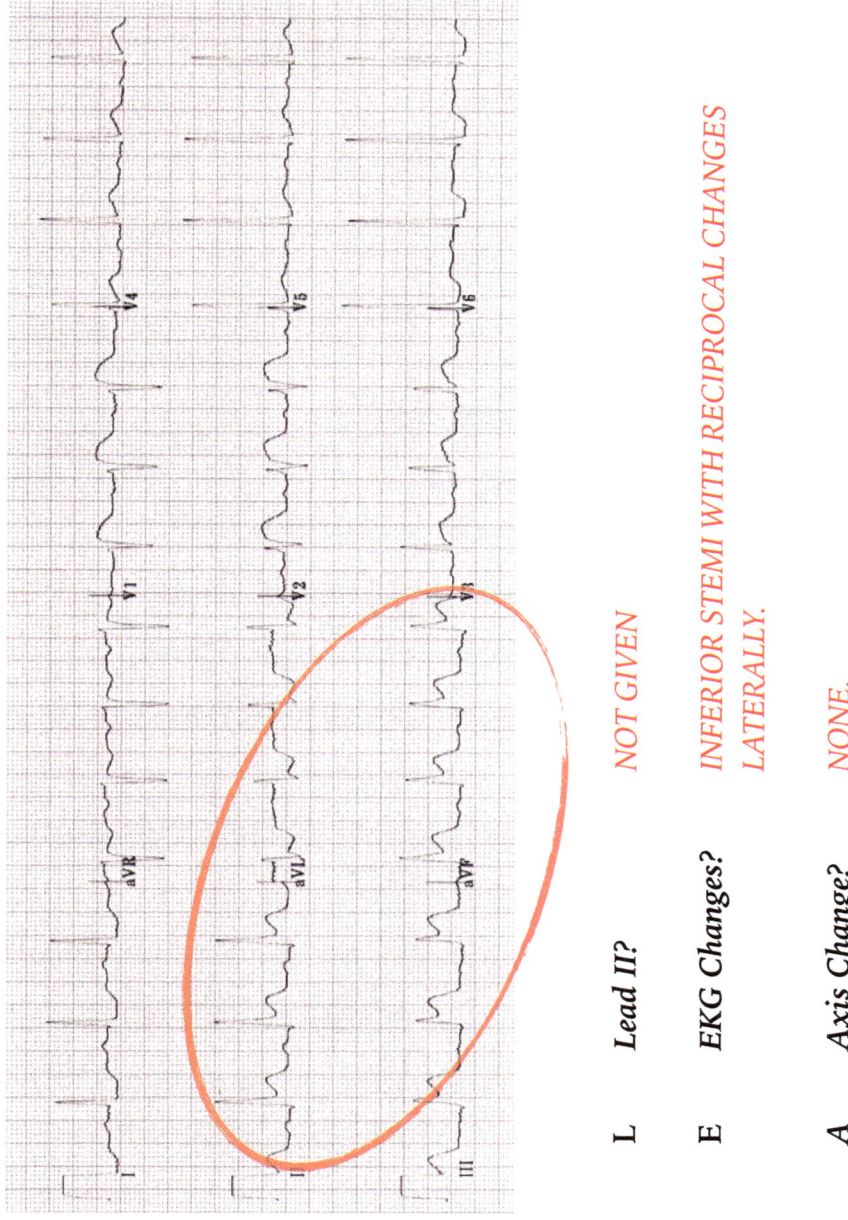

- **L**   *Lead II?*   NOT GIVEN
- **E**   *EKG Changes?*   INFERIOR STEMI WITH RECIPROCAL CHANGES LATERALLY.
- **A**   *Axis Change?*   NONE.
- **D**   *Differentials?*   POTENTIAL FOR RIGHT VENTRICULAR.
- **S**   *Stability?*   CURRENTLY STABLE, YET REQUIRES RAPID TRANSPORT TO A CARDIAC CARE CENTER.

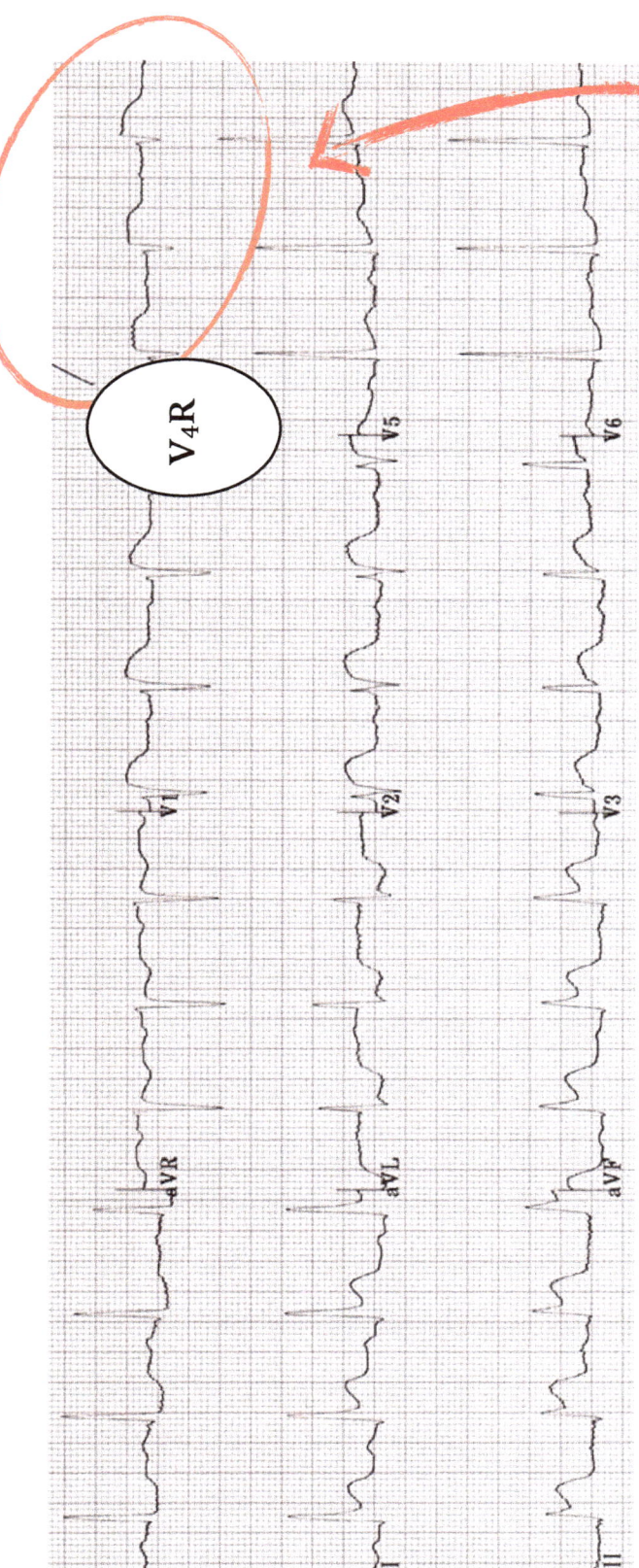

V₄R

CONFIRMED RIGHT VENTRICULAR INVOLVEMENT

REMEMBER: 500ml BOLUS BEFORE NITROGLYCERIN ADMINISTRATION

EKG #5

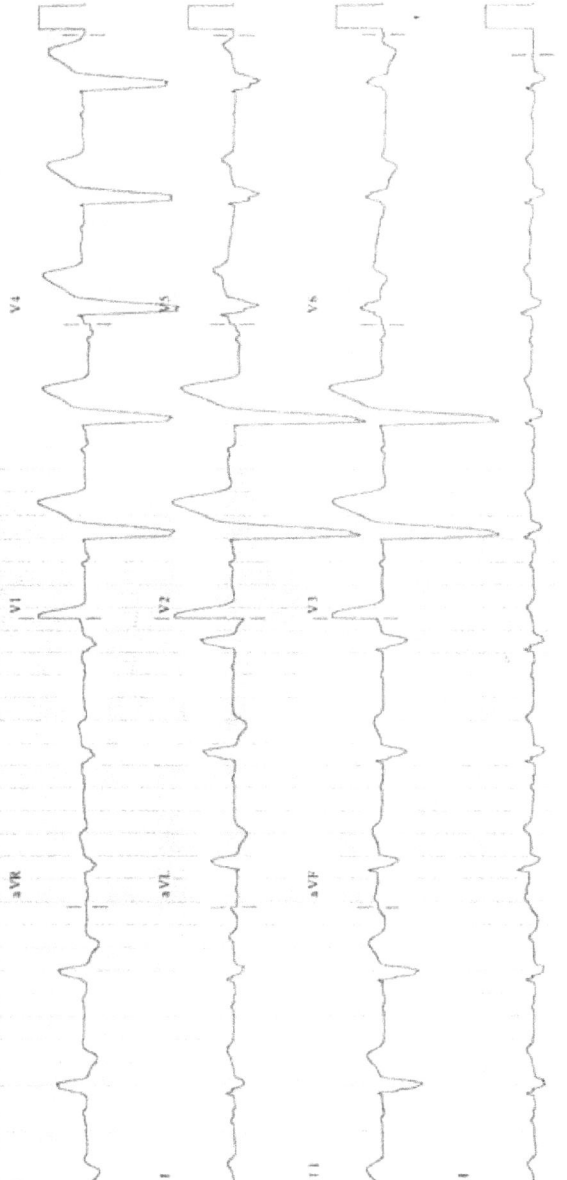

EKG from litfl.com

You arrive on scene to find a 48-year-old, intoxicated male sitting in his car and complaining of shortness of breath and chest pressure for one day. He has a history of cirrhosis and methamphetamine use, yet denies ever having any heart problems. He denies meth use today and states he doesn't take any medications. His vital signs are: blood pressure 188/80; heart rate of 80; respirations of 28 and saturations of 99%. He's alert and oriented, pale, cool, and moist; his lungs are clear bilaterally; his abdomen is without pulsating mass; his pulses are equal and he has no peripheral edema.

L   *Lead II?* _____

E   *EKG Changes?* _____

A   *Axis Change?* _____

D   *Differentials?* _____

S   *Stability?* _____

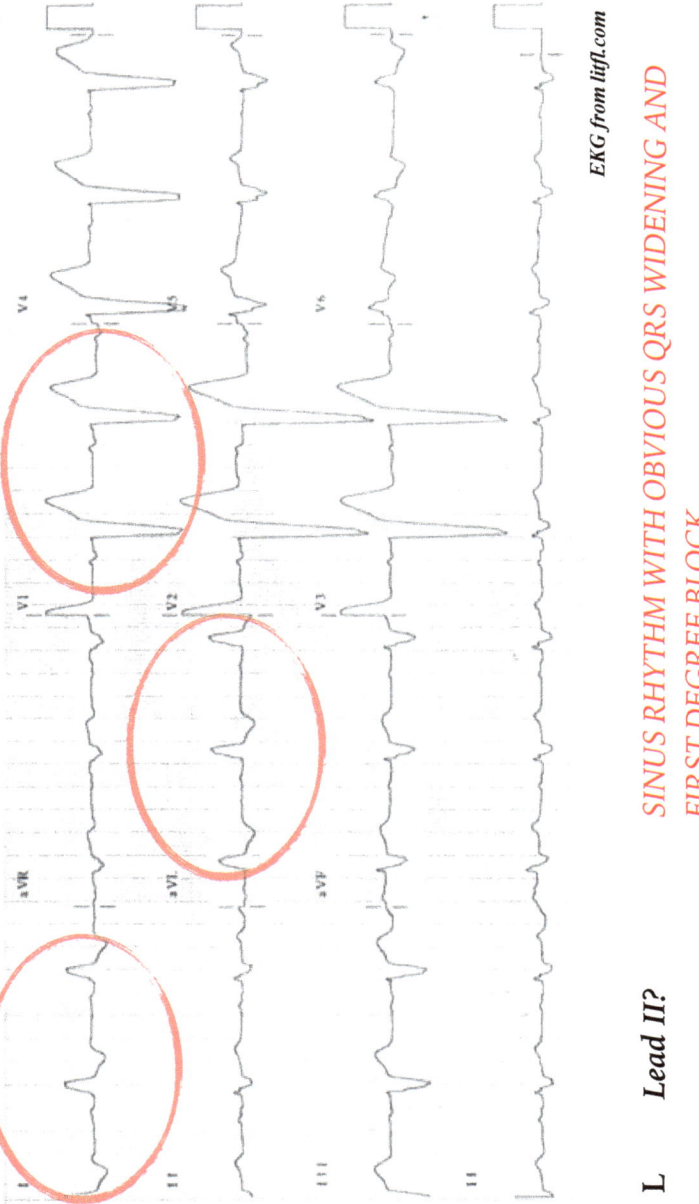

EKG from litfl.com

L   *Lead II?*   SINUS RHYTHM WITH OBVIOUS QRS WIDENING AND FIRST DEGREE BLOCK.

E   *EKG Changes?*   UNABLE TO INTERPRET DUE TO WIDENED QRS WIDTH.

A   *Axis Change?*   LEFT AXIS DEVIATION WITH WIDENED QRS >1.2mm DIAGNOSTIC FOR LBBB.

D   *Differentials?*   HIGH POTENTIAL FOR UNDERLYING STEMI DUE TO EKG, DRUG USE, PRESENTATION, AND LACK OF KNOWN CARDIAC HISTORY. CONSIDER PE, ENDOCARDITIS, TAA, AND PNEUMOTHORAX.

S   *Stability?*   CURRENTLY STABLE, YET TRANSPORT QUICKLY.

EKG #6

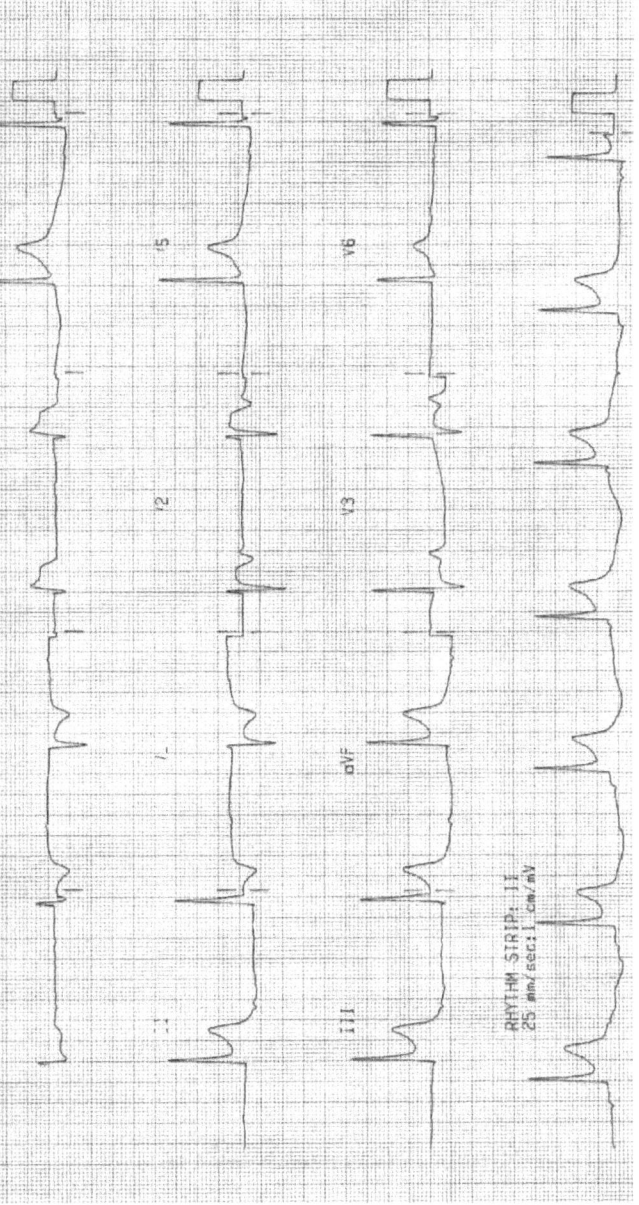

EKG from litfl.com

You arrive on scene to find a 89-year-old female complaining of weakness for two days. Family states that she will not get out of bed. She has a history of Alzheimer's, hypertension, and hypothyroid. Family is trying to find her medication list. Her vital signs are: blood pressure of 74/60; heart rate of 50; respirations 16; saturations of 95%. She's groggy, but alert to her norm; she's pink, warm, and dry; her pupils are equal and reactive; her lungs are clear and equal; her abdomen is soft and non-tender; she has 2⁺, non-pitting edema to both ankles and equal, bilateral pedal and radial pulses. She doesn't have a DNR.

L   Lead II? _____

E   EKG Changes? _____

A   Axis Change? _____

D   Differentials? _____

S   Stability? _____

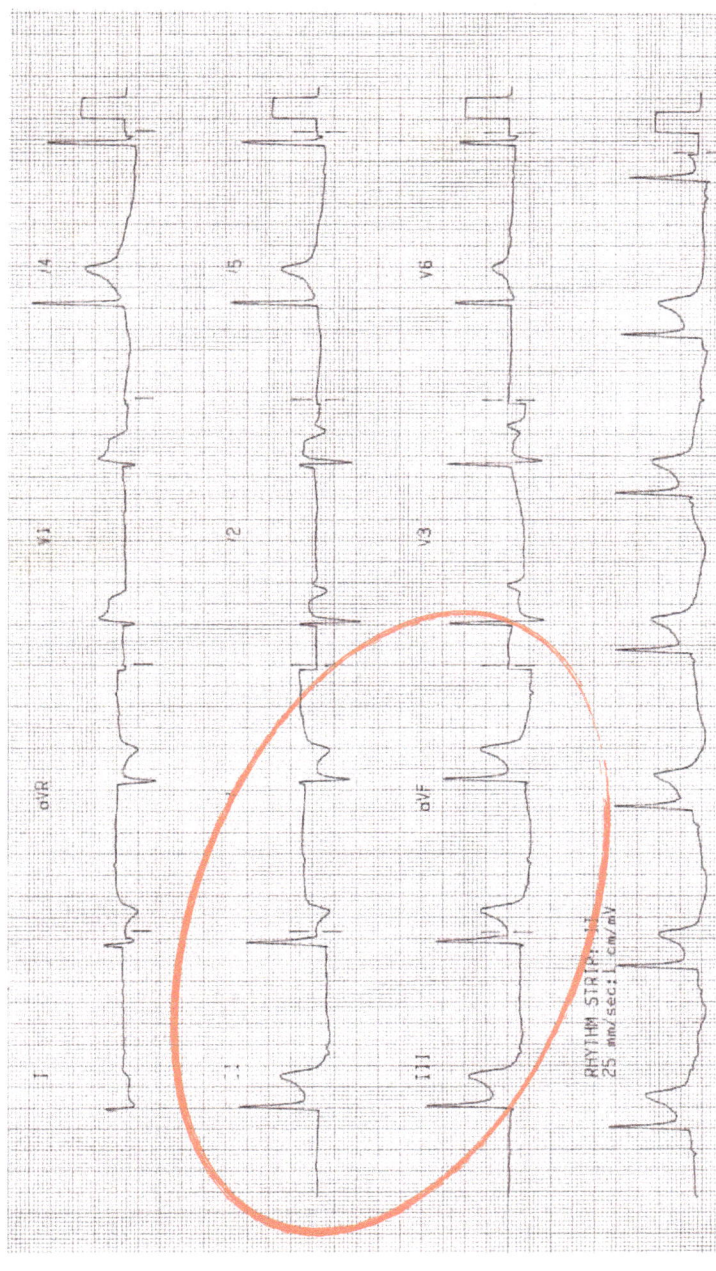

EKG from litfl.com

L   *Lead II?*   SINUS BRADYCARDIA WITH FIRST DEGREE BLOCK AND OBVIOUS ST ELEVATION (CONSIDER HYDRATION, ATROPINE, PACING DUE TO HYPOTENSION).

E   *EKG Changes?*   INFERIOR STEMI (CONSIDER RV INVOLVEMENT) WITH RECIPROCAL CHANGES TO THE HIGH LATERAL LEADS. ST ELEVATION ALSO NOTED TO THE SEPTAL LEADS.

A   *Axis Change?*   NO.

D   *Differentials?*   NO, THE DIAGNOSIS IS CLEAR.

S   *Stability?*   HYPOTENSION AND LOW HEART RATE IS CONCERNING. HIGH LIKELIHOOD OF DETERIORATION.

EKG #7

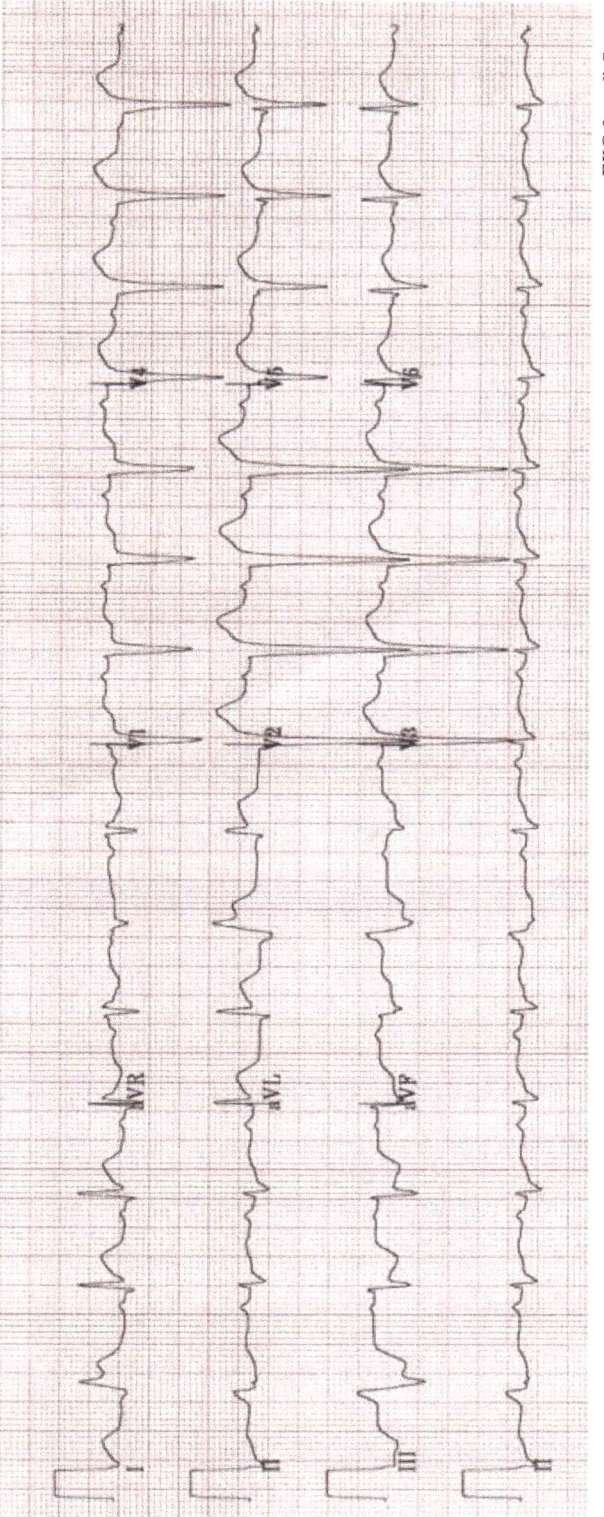

EKG from litfl.com

You arrive on scene to find a 69-year-old male complaining of chest *"burning"* for one day. He states it awoke him from his nap yesterday. Thinking it was heartburn, he took four Tums® without relief. He has a history of GERD. He only takes Protonix®. His vital signs are: blood pressure of 102/60; heart rate of 86; respirations of 16; saturations of 98%. He's alert and oriented; he's pink, warm, and dry; his pupils are equal and reactive; his lungs are clear and equal; his abdomen is soft and non-tender. He has no edema to note and he has equal, bilateral pulses to his pedal and radial pulses.

L   *Lead II?* _____

E   *EKG Changes?* _____

A   *Axis Change?* _____

D   *Differentials?* _____

S   *Stability?* _____

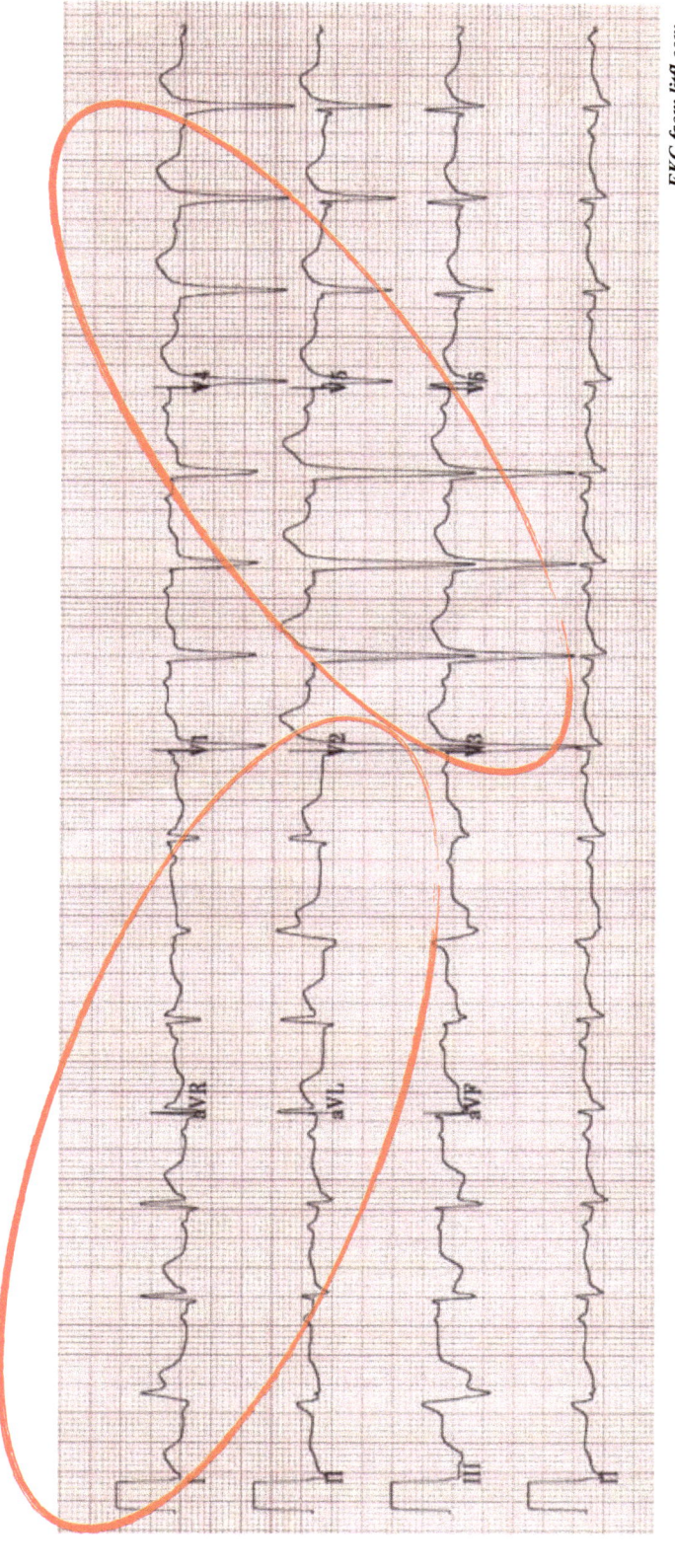

EKG from litfl.com

L Lead II?   SINUS RHYTHM WITH POTENTIAL ST DEPRESSION.

E EKG Changes?   ST ELEVATION TO THE HIGH LATERAL AND ANTERIOR LEADS WITH RECIPROCAL CHANGES INFERIORLY.

A Axis Change?   LEFT.

D Differentials? CLEAR DIAGNOSIS OF STEMI.

S Stability?   STABLE CURRENTLY. RAPID TRANSPORT ADVISED.

EKG #8

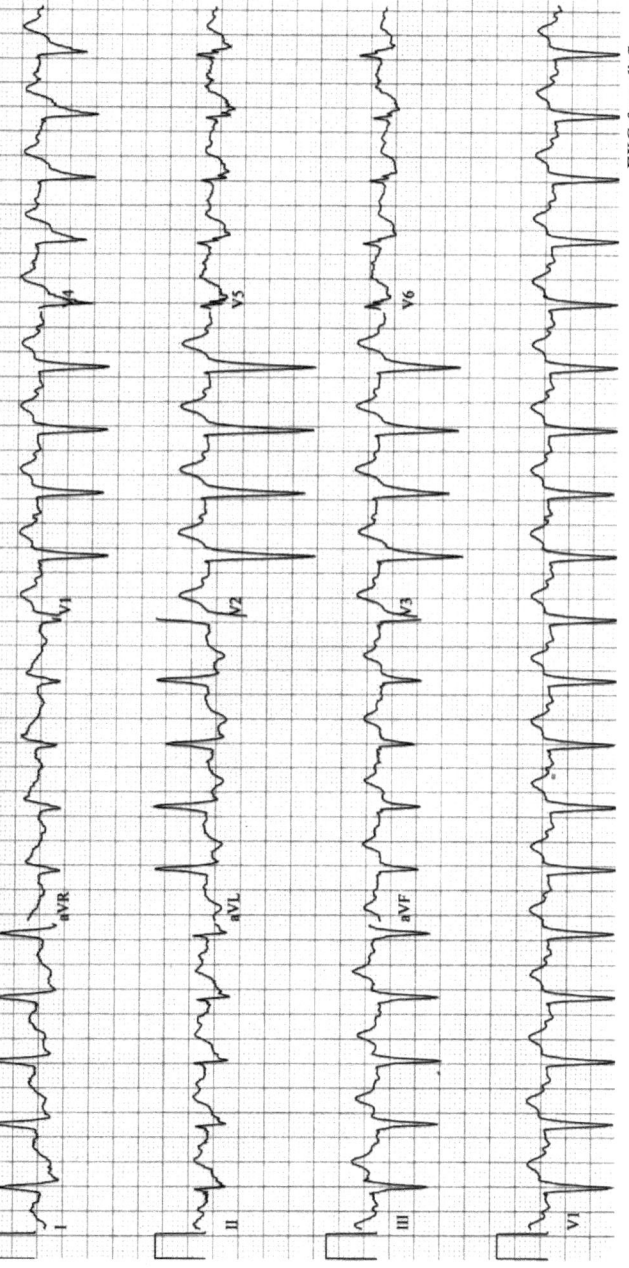

EKG from litfl.com

You arrive on scene to find a 41-year-old, morbidly obese male complaining of chest pain for six hours. He states his pain began after an argument with his mother. He has a history of an MI three years ago and today's symptoms, *"Feel the same."* His history includes GERD, insulin-dependent diabetes, hypertension, hypercholesterolemia, and sleep apnea. When asked about his medications, he states *"I take something for diabetes and some other stuff."* He does not know where his medications are. His vital signs are: blood pressure of 168/80; heart rate of 104; respirations of 30; saturations of 98%. He's alert and oriented; he's diaphoretic; his pupils are equal and reactive; his lungs reveal bilateral crackles; his abdomen is distended, yet soft and non-tender; There's significant peripheral edema noted, but he has equal, bilateral pulses to his pedal and radial pulses.

L   Lead II? _____

E   EKG Changes? _____

A   Axis Change? _____

D   Differentials? _____

S   Stability? _____

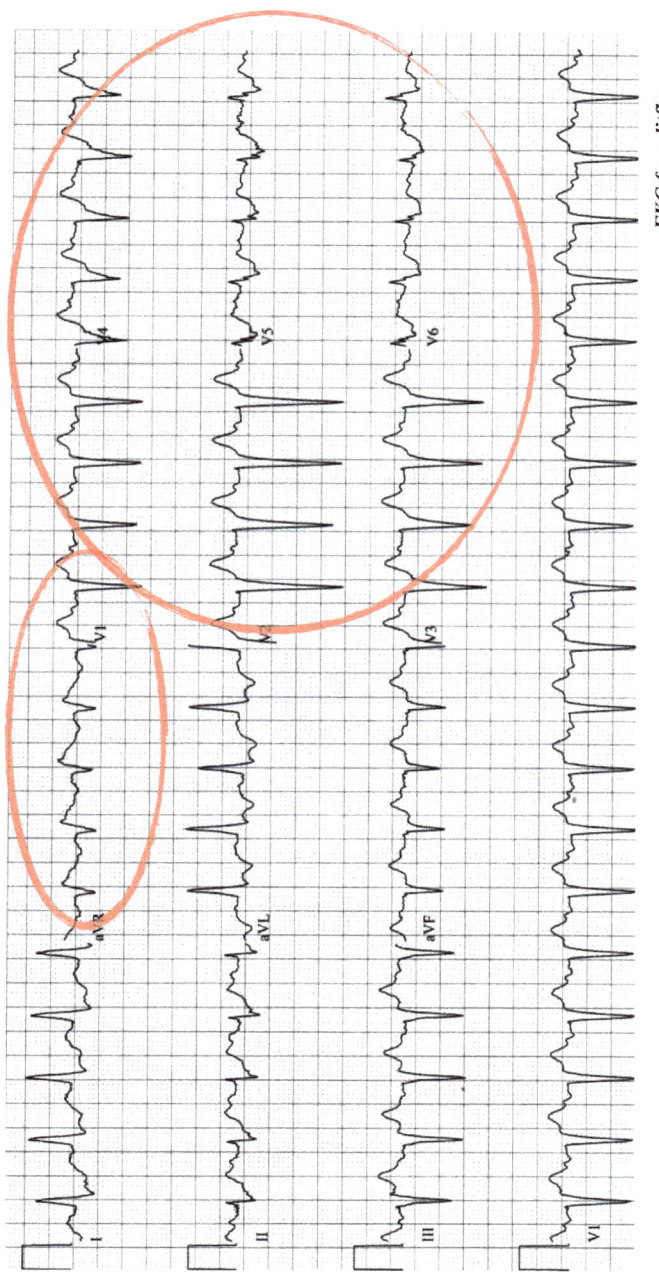

EKG from litfl.com

L   *Lead II?*   SINUS TACHYCARDIA.

E   *EKG Changes?*   DIFFUSE ST DEPRESSION ACROSS THE PRECORDIAL LEADS WITH ST ELEVATION IN aVR.

A   *Axis Change?*   LEFT AXIS DEVIATION, YET QRS REMAINS <1.2mm.

D   *Differentials?*   CONCERN FOR POTENTIAL LMCA OCCLUSION DUE TO ST ELEVATION IN aVR WITH DIFFUSE PRECORDIAL ST DEPRESSION.

S   *Stability?*   HIGH POTENTIAL FOR ARREST DUE TO COMPLETE ISCHEMIA TO THE LEFT VENTRICLE.

EKG #9

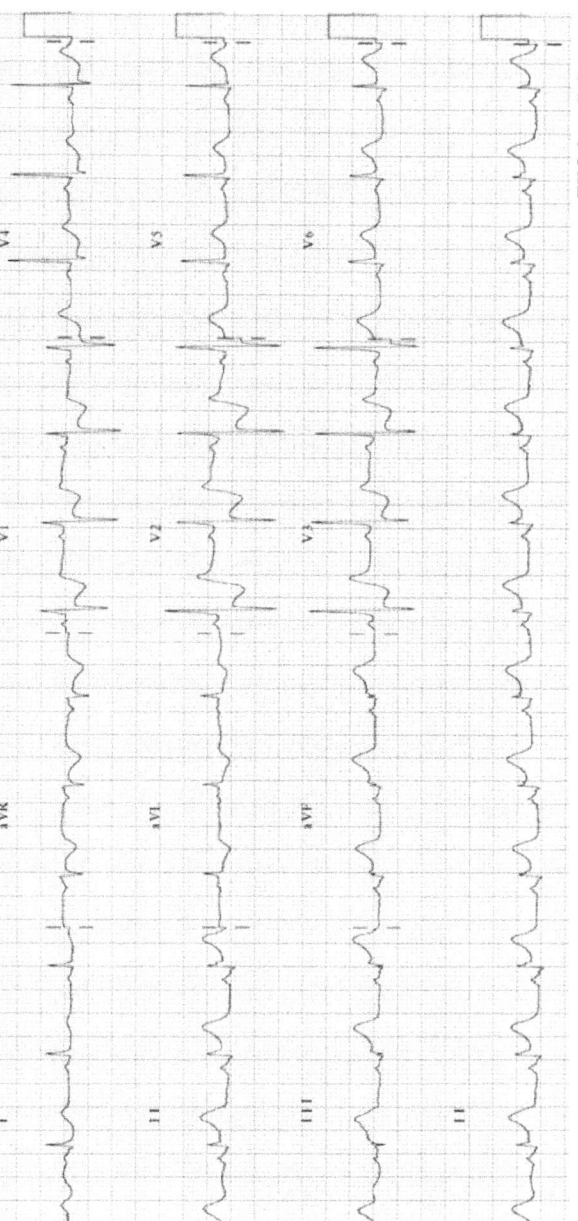

EKG from litfl.com

You arrive on scene to find a 53-year-old female complaining of *"not feeling right"* for 30 minutes. She states her symptoms came on rapidly while doing the dishes and she had to sit down in order to keep from "throwing up." She has a history of hypothyroid, fibromyalgia, and migraines. She takes Elavil, levothyroxine, and Topomax®. Her vital signs are: blood pressure of 200/90; heart rate of 98; respirations of 24; saturations of 98%. She's alert and oriented. She's diaphoretic; her pupils equal and reactive; her lungs are clear; her abdomen is benign. She has no edema to note and she has equal, bilateral pedal and radial pulses.

L   *Lead II?*   _____

E   *EKG Changes?*   _____

A   *Axis Change?*   _____

D   *Differentials?*   _____

S   *Stability?*   _____

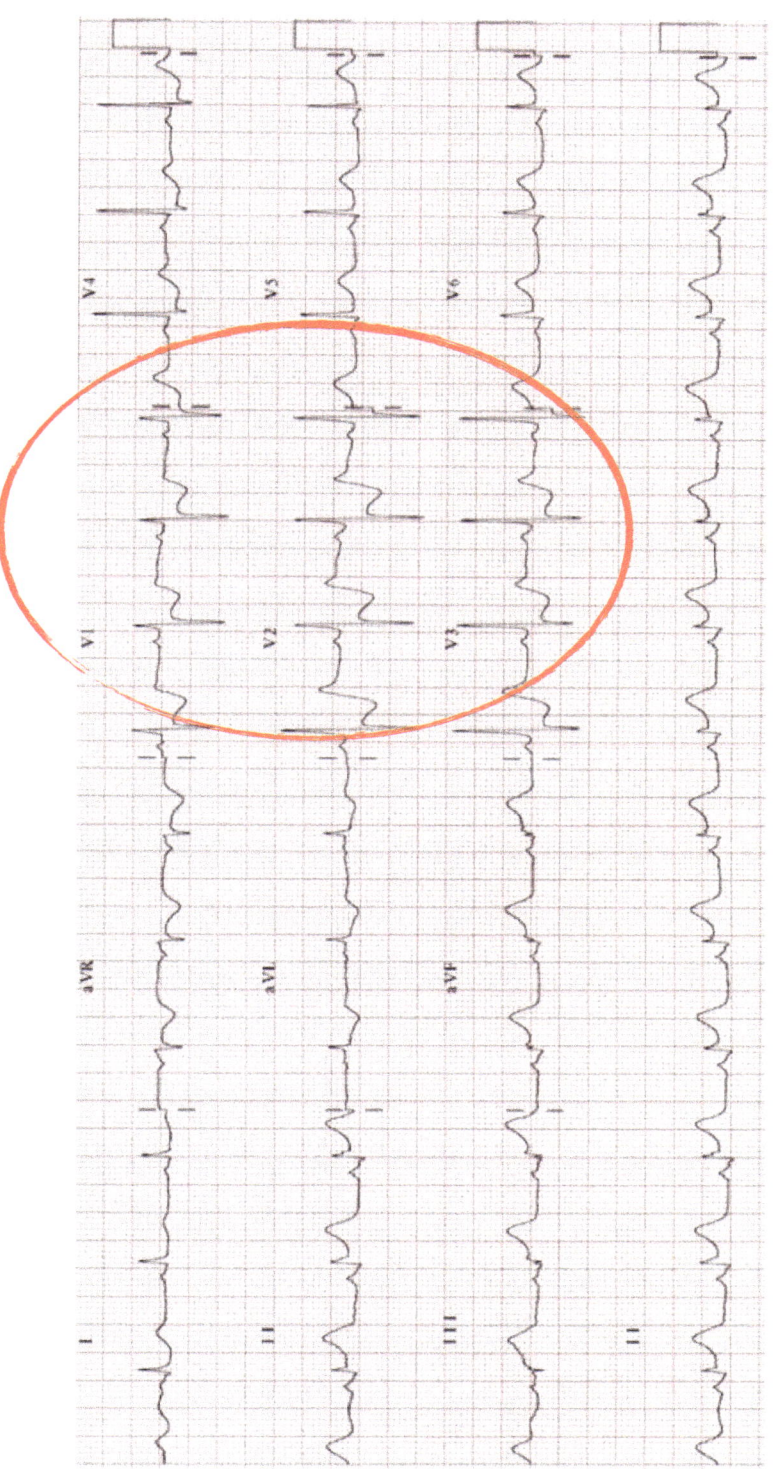

L	Lead II?	SINUS RHYTHM WITH OBVIOUS INFERIOR ST ELEVATION.
E	EKG Changes?	INFERIOR STEMI WITH RECIPROCAL CHANGE TO THE SEPTAL AND ANTERIOR LEADS.
A	Axis Change?	NO.
D	Differentials?	POTENTIAL FOR A POSTERIOR MI.
S	Stability?	AT RISK FOR RAPID DETERIORATION.

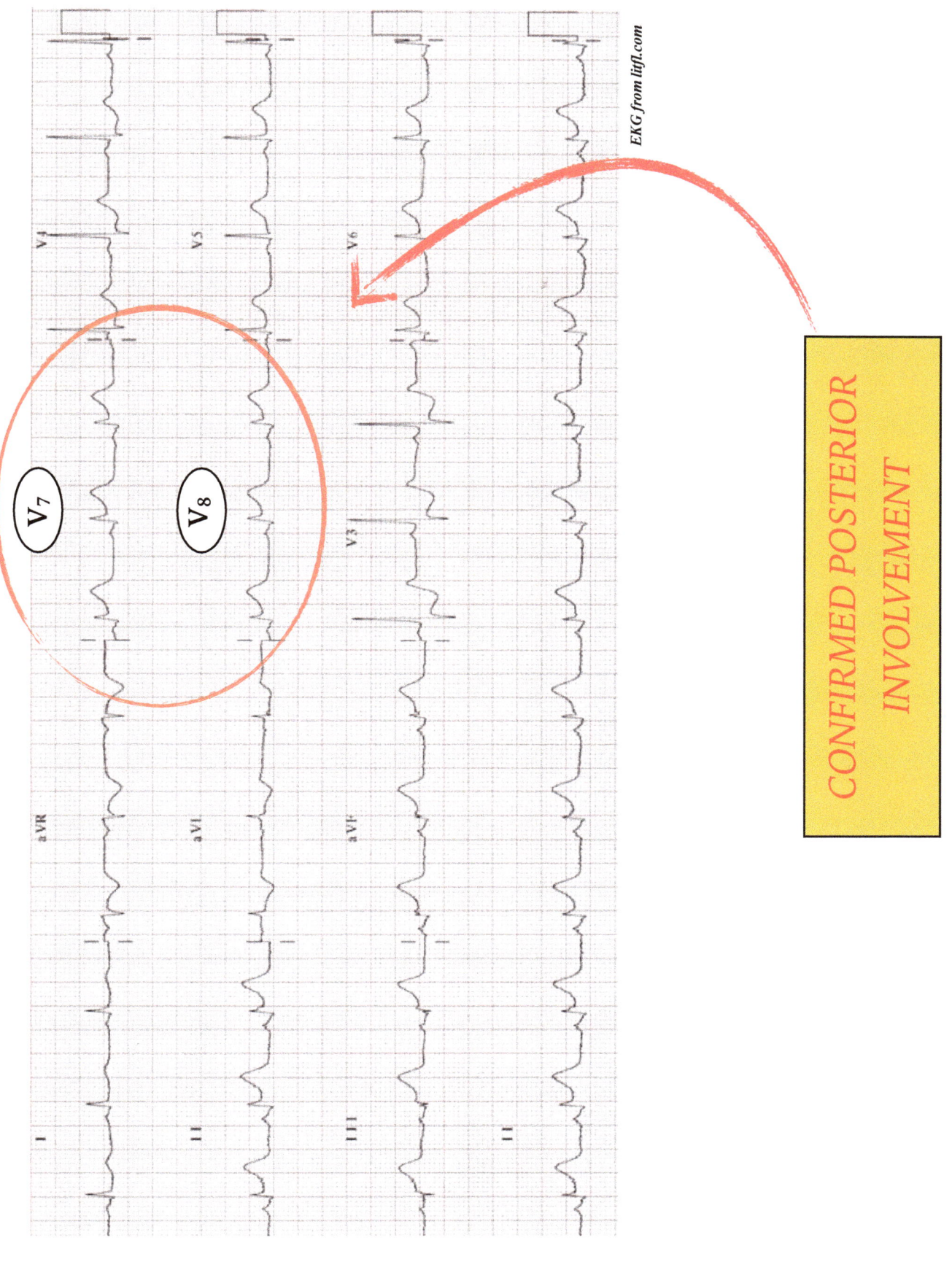

EKG #10

EKG from litfl.com

You arrive on scene to find a 76-year-old female complaining of increasing dizziness for two days. She states she can't stand without *"passing out."* She has a history of hypertension and takes metoprolol. Her vital signs are: blood pressure 68/p; heart rate between 20-30; respirations 20; sats 98%. She's confused and ashen; her pupils are equal and reactive; her lungs are clear; her abdomen is benign; no edema is noted and she has equal, bilateral pulses to the pedal and radial pulses.

L *Lead II?* _____

E *EKG Changes?* N/A

A *Axis Change?* N/A

D *Differentials?* _____

S *Stability?* _____

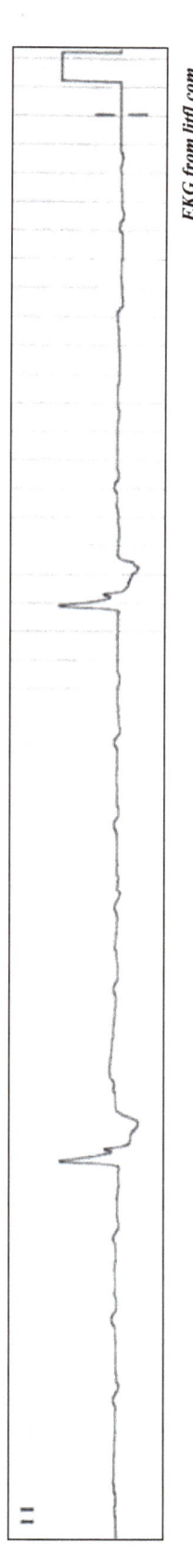

EKG from litfl.com

L *Lead II?* SIGNIFICANT BRADYCARDIA WITH COMPLETE HEART BLOCK.

E *EKG Changes?* N/A.

A *Axis Change?* N/A.

D *Differentials?* MYOCARDIAL INFARCTION VS BETA-BLOCKER OVERDOSE VS NEUROLOGIC VS OTHER.

S *Stability?* UNSTABLE. VERY HIGH RISK FOR ARREST.

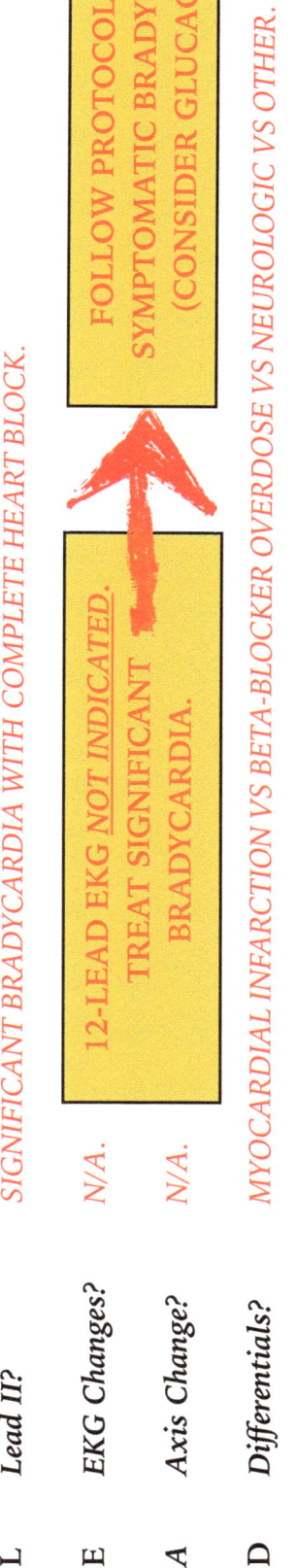

12-LEAD EKG *NOT INDICATED.* TREAT SIGNIFICANT BRADYCARDIA.

FOLLOW PROTOCOLS FOR SYMPTOMATIC BRADYCARDIA (CONSIDER GLUCAGON)

7

Calling the Hospital with a Cardiac Patient: The Dos and *Don'ts*

With each lecture it's inevitable that an astute student will ask how they accurately communicate their EKG findings to the hospital. This is an important question, for prehospital information is useless if the receiving hospital cannot understand it. A lack of ability to deliver a clear, succinct report will prompt unnecessary questions from the hospital staff that will subsequently delay care. This chapter provides some essential tips to effectively relay your findings, including some examples of the dos and don'ts I've learned and taught over the years.

Slow Down

First and foremost, slow down. It's all too routine for field personnel to speak very quickly when giving report. Rapid-fire reporting is often due a nervousness about being on the spot; the quicker I can get it over with, the better. Keep in mind that the hospital staff is often dealing with numerous other tasks while they try to decipher what you're saying, and slowing down your report gives them ample time to discern and scribe what you're conveying. Firing off your report only leads to more questions, more time on the radio, and less time treating the patient in front of you.

Keep It Simple

It's paramount to keep your report *simple*. Never attempt to woo your audience with superfluous or esoteric findings; they don't care about irrelevant information, and, in all likelihood, won't take you seriously if you offer it. So you did a 12-lead on a patient with congestive heart failure and knew how to identify a ventricular strain pattern (not addressed in this text)—great—yet this information is irrelevant. Your receiving hospital only wants to know if there is an *immediate* need (i.e., calling the cardiologist/

catheterization team or preparing for an impending arrest). Here are examples of dos and a don'ts when relaying your radio report.

> DON'T: *On board I have a 46-year-old male complaining of shortness of breath and chest pain for three days. He has no significant history. His vitals are stable and the 12-lead EKG reveals a sinus tachycardia at 104 with $S_1Q_3T_3$ changes. Our ETA is six minutes.*

Ok. It was impressive that this paramedic knew the $S_1Q_3T_3$ pattern, which can be suggestive of a *possible* pulmonary embolism. While differentials are essential to successful prehospital practice, this finding doesn't need to be dealt with promptly, or told to the hospital during your radio report. *Are there any arrhythmias or ST changes?* That's what they want to know. Any other findings can be given at bedside. A simple approach is more respected and appreciated. Here's a good example of a concise report involving the same patient.

> DO: *On board is a 46-year-old male complaining of shortness of breath and chest pain for three days. He has no significant history. His vitals are stable and the <u>12-lead EKG reveals no obvious ST change</u>. I am following ALS protocols and our ETA is six minutes.*

This report is succinct, professional, and well organized. This patient doesn't need immediate intervention, and that important detail was conveyed effectively.

Know What You're Talking About and Get to the Point

You should always know what you're talking about and get to the point quickly. Don't give vague interpretations or esoteric findings. It's most useful when you can tell the receiving hospital precisely what's going on in as few words as possible: this is what this patient has, this is what I did about it, and this is what this patient needs. Skip the non-pertinent details. The following page contains some examples.

DO: *En route to you, Code 3, with a STEMI activation on a 60-year-old female complaining of chest pain for one hour. She's hypertensive at 170/90 and bradycardic at 50. The 12-lead shows an inferior STEMI with no evidence of right-right-sided involvement. We are ALS. Our ETA is four minutes.*

Perfect! There's no need to say, *"ST changes in leads II, III, and aVF"* or *"reciprocal changes in the lateral leads."* They know it's a STEMI and likely know which leads are the inferior leads. Here is what the receiving hospital might get out of this:

1. EMS is coming in quickly and I need to get ready.
2. It's a STEMI activation: Call the cath lab.
3. Vital signs are hemodynamically stable: There's no need for immediate stabilization.
4. It's an inferior STEMI without right-sided involvement: This is pertinent for the cardiologist on call, although not necessarily pertinent as EMS told me it was a STEMI activation.
5. EMS is following ALS protocols: IV, aspirin, etc. If EMS skipped something or couldn't get an IV, they would've mentioned it (always mention skipped steps or that which you didn't do).
6. Their ETA is four minutes: This is how much time I have to prepare.

Straightforward. Done. This paramedic knows what a cardiac patient looks like and what the course of action should be. The hospital is now ready to receive this patient.

DON'T: *En route to you with a 60-year-old female complaining of chest pain for one hour. She states her pain is substernal, radiating to her left shoulder and described as "squeezing." She has a history of insulin dependent diabetes and hypertension. She takes Levemir and Humolog along with Lisinopril, of which she missed her dose. She is hypertensive at 172/90, bradycardic at 50 and has a respiratory rate of 12 with saturations of 95%. The 12-lead shows a STEMI. She is on oxygen at 15 liters per minute with an IV placed. She has received one spray of nitroglycerin and four 81 milligram aspirin. Our ETA is now 30 seconds. This is a STEMI activation.*

This report was longwinded and filled with superfluous information. Organized and condensed reports are the most effective means to convey information because they leave little question. Here's what the hospital might have gained from this report—if they didn't walk away from the radio:

1. The patient has chest pain.
2. They take several medications, *"I think for diabetes."* Were the vitals stable?
3. They did a 12-lead, right?
4. *"Wait, what?! It's a STEMI!?"*
5. *"30 seconds! I have no time to prepare to receive this patient! All my beds are full!"*

Think about the person having to write all this down. He or she may have numerous other ambulances coming in, two admissions, and lost lab results to track down, etc. A paramedic friend of mine wisely told me that report giving is just like writing a newspaper article; you've got two sentences to grab your audience because that's all they hear anyway. Finally, the less time you talk, the more time the receiving hospital must prepare for your arrival and you to care for your patient.

Know Your Protocols

Protocols are essential. Never just wing it or go cowboy, as they say. Some EMS areas require two millimeters of ST change in two adjoining leads, others one millimeter of ST change. If you don't know or follow your regions established protocol, how can you be trusted? You'll be seen as incompetent and put your patient in jeopardy, raising legal concerns that would negatively effect your license.

Be Confident and Stand Your Ground

Stick to your guns. Confidence takes time to develop, yet if you're looking at your patient and the EKG and you see a STEMI (however, small), call it. Make a choice and stick with it. Erring on the side of caution is never wrong. Don't say, *"maybe"* or *"possible STEMI."* Does the EKG meet criteria or doesn't it? Have you used your practiced pattern to diagnose?

DON'T: *En route with a possible non-STEMI on a 41-year-old female complaining of shortness of breath. Vitals are within normal limits, yet she has T-wave changes in V_{1-4}.*

There are two mistakes to note here:

1. Generally, receiving hospitals don't care much about *NSTEMIs,* as they require cardiac lab work to fully identify. This said, it doesn't mean you should not speak up, or transport accordingly. Finally, avoid the use of the word, *possible;* is it or isn't it?
2. *T-wave changes* will prompt the question, *"What changes?"* In this case, relay that you have *ischemic changes.*

NSTEMI findings may cause a push back by emergency department staff depending on the facility's capabilities. However, they don't see what you see—the EKG and the patient—and you don't have all the diagnostic instruments that the receiving facility has at their disposal, so stand your ground. Stick to your guns if you believe you've come to the right course of action. If it turns out to be something other than what you thought, look at the situation as a learning experience.

Often, hospital staff assume that you don't know anything, and this is true in many areas, for ALS personnel aren't comfortable with the information the 12-lead provides. A prehospital provider's duty is to treat their patient to the best of their ability and training—and to subtlety prove hospital doubters wrong, thus propping up the profession.

Don't Take Criticism Too Personally

Don't beat yourself up when you make mistakes and don't make excuses for your errors. Mistakes are inevitable, yet they aid in further learning; you can't learn if you're never wrong. Whenever you hear a colleague say, *"I would've gotten the tube if my partner had checked out the ambulance this morning and stocked a 7.5,"* or *"I would've cardioverted them but I didn't want to restock the narcs,"* it's because they either screwed up or were so unsure of what they were doing that they're defensive and making excuses. So, be professional and sincere. Step up when you screwed up and ask for feedback so you can improve.

Get Feedback

Inviting feedback and criticism into your career is the best way to learn and grow. Knowing what and how to do better is the only way to improve. People who only listen to or seek out those who continually tell them they're amazing learn nothing. Here are some possible questions that you may want to ask the receiving hospital staff after delivering a patient:

1. *Did I provide too much or too little information in my report?*
2. *How was the organization of the information given?*
3. *Do you have any suggestions that could make my report better or more useful?*

Here are some additional questions you may want to ask the receiving physician:

1. *Was my treatment appropriate?*
2. *Was my interpretation of the 12-lead EKG correct?*
3. *How was my bedside report?*
4. *Do you have any suggestions on how I could improve?*
5. *What are you going to do next for the patient?*

That last question is critical to your learning. It allows you to know the flow as well as gives you an idea of the fruits of your labor. Ask if you can continue to observe if they (or you) aren't too busy.

Don't be dissuaded if you're brushed off the first few times; the staff may be too busy or are simply having a bad day. Don't take it personally. It happens to us all. I've blown students off due to fatigue or other work or life frustrations, and it was nothing about them; I was just not in the right frame of mind to instruct. In this case, ask the emergency department staff to be on the lookout for anything you could improve upon in the future, and if their disinterest continues, find someone else, especially the receiving physician. Most medical professionals are willing to provide suggestion, as many were involved in EMS in their past.

Asking for critique shows humility and a willingness to better yourself. Humility is something very often lost in medicine. There's not a person, no matter their level of training, from whom you cannot learn. Also, remember that placing your betterment above your ego also improves care for your patients and makes the hospital's job easier in the long run, making them appreciate you more.

These are just a few topics that I've found influential to my career when addressing the transfer of care to the hospital staff. The point of this chapter was to encourage your development and confidence with each patient that you see. Don't look at the hospital as a safe zone to dump your patient because you were not comfortable with a needed procedure or medication. Do the procedure, give the medication when appropriate, and remember the Hippocratic Oath: *"Do No Harm."* Performance is the only way to learn and better yourself. Such proactivity will also build the confidence of the hospital staff toward you. If you try and your treatment doesn't go as planned, cop up to your mistakes and learn from them. There's not a medical professional out there who hasn't made mistakes, including myself. If you practice and learn during your career, you'll begin to treat patients efficiently and accurately, and your confidence will shine through.

Takeaway Notes from Chapter 7:

- *Slow down when you speak on the radio.*

- *Keep it simple! Everything is clearer and easier to deal with if you just keep it simple. Don't overthink and don't regurgitate erroneous information over the radio.*

- *Know what you're talking about! Never wing it or make it up. Study and grow. This helps ease your anxiety as well as increase the receiving hospital's confidence in you.*

- *Know your protocols!*

- *Be confident in what you say and stand your ground! Don't let others walk over you if you believe you made the right decision. Most of the time the one criticizing is just grandstanding anyway.*

- *Don't take criticisms too personally. Listen to what they have to say, no matter their tone; sift through the information and take home anything you can try in the future—try to forget the rest.*

Get Feedback. This is important, especially when speaking to the ER physician regarding an unstable case you delivered. This will better your practice in the end. If possible, find someone who's willing to mentor you. This is a productive way to build relationships, network, and grow—and you might find that you have something to offer them as well.

Acronym Glossary

ACS	Acute coronary syndrome
AV	Atrioventricular node
aVR	Atrioventricular right
aVL	Atrioventricular left
aVF	Atrioventricular foot
EKG	Electrocardiogram
EMT	Emergency Medical Technician
ETA	Estimated time of arrival
IV	Intravenous catheter
LAD	Left anterior descending artery
LBBB	Left bundle branch block
LCx	Left circumflex artery
LMCA	Left main coronary artery
RCA	Right coronary artery
MI	Myocardial infarction
MONA	Morphine, oxygen, nitroglycerin, aspirin
NSTEMI	Non-ST-elevation myocardial infarction
PVC	Premature ventricular complex
RBBB	Right bundle branch block
SA	Sino-atrial node
STEMI	ST-elevation myocardial infarction
V_4R	Ventricular 4, right (Right precordial lead)

References

Chapter 1

Burns, Edward. (2007). *Normal 12-Lead EKG*. Retrieved from https://lifeinthefastlane.com (assessed February 8, 2017).

Chapter 2

Burns, Edward. (2007). *Anterio-lateral STEMI*. Retrieved from https://lifeinthefastlane.com (assessed March 19, 2017).

Burns, Edward. (2007). *Inferior STEMI*. Retrieved from https://lifeinthefastlane.com (assessed March 19, 2017).

Burns, Edward. (2007). *Inferior Q Waves*. Retrieved from https://lifeinthefastlane.com (assessed March 19, 2017).

Chapter 3

Burns, Edward. (2007). *Normal 12-Lead EKG*. Retrieved from https://lifeinthefastlane.com (assessed January 17, 2017).

Burns, Edward. (2007). *Septo-anterior STEMI*. Retrieved from https://lifeinthefastlane.com (assessed January 17, 2017).

Burns, Edward. (2007). *High lateral STEMI*. Retrieved from https://lifeinthefastlane.com (assessed January 17, 2017).

Burns, Edward. (2007). *Left main coronary infarct*. Retrieved from https://lifeinthefastlane.com (assessed February 10, 2018).

Burns, Edward. (2007). *Inferior STEMI*. Retrieved from https://lifeinthefastlane.com (assessed February 10, 2018).

Burns, Edward. (2007). *Inferior STEMI with posterior changes*. Retrieved from https://lifeinthefastlane.com (assessed February 10, 2018).

Chapter 3 *(Continued)*

Burns, Edward. (2007). *Inferior STEMI with reciprocal change.* Retrieved from https://lifeinthefastlane.com (assessed February 10, 2018).

Burns, Edward. (2007). *Inferior STEMI with right sided infarction.* Retrieved from https://lifeinthefastlane.com (assessed February 10, 2018).

Burns, Edward. (2007). *Posterior STEMI.* Retrieved from https://lifeinthefastlane.com (assessed February 10, 2018).

Burns, Edward. (2007). *Proximal LAD occlusion.* Retrieved from https://lifeinthefastlane.com (assessed February 10, 2018).

Chapter 4

Burns, Edward. (2007). *Normal QRS axis.* Retrieved from https://lifeinthefastlane.com (assessed February 10, 2018).

Burns, Edward. (2007). *Left axis deviation.* Retrieved from https://lifeinthefastlane.com (assessed March 19, 2018).

Burns, Edward. (2007). *Left bundle branch block.* Retrieved from https://lifeinthefastlane.com (assessed February 10, 2018).

Burns, Edward. (2007). *Right axis deviation.* Retrieved from https://lifeinthefastlane.com (assessed February 10, 2018).

Burns, Edward. (2007). *Sinus rhythm with unifocal PVC.* Retrieved from https://lifeinthefastlane.com (assessed March 19, 2018).

Chapter 5

Burns, Edward. (2007). *Anterior-septal STEMI with lateral involvement.* Retrieved from https://lifeinthefastlane.com (assessed February 10, 2018).

Burns, Edward. (2007). *Inferior STEMI with lateral reciprocal changes.* Retrieved from https://lifeinthefastlane.com (assessed January 14, 2018).

Chapter 5 *(Continued)*

Burns, Edward. (2007). *Lateral NSTEMI.* Retrieved from https://lifeinthefastlane.com (assessed May 20, 2018).

Burns, Edward. (2007). *Left bundle branch block.* Retrieved from https://lifeinthefastlane.com (assessed May 20, 2018).

Burns, Edward. (2007). *Normal sinus rhythm with widened QRS interval.* Retrieved from https://lifeinthefastlane.com (assessed May 20, 2018).

Burns, Edward. (2007). *Anterio-septal STEMI with inferior reciprocal change.* Retrieved from https://lifeinthefastlane.com (assessed January 31st, 2019).

Burns, Edward. (2007). *Inferior STEMI with reciprocal change.* Retrieved from https://lifeinthefastlane.com (assessed January 31st, 2019).

Burns, Edward. (2007). *Right sided STEMI shown in V_4R.* Retrieved from https://lifeinthefastlane.com (assessed May 20, 2018).

Burns, Edward. (2007). *Sinus arrhythmia.* Retrieved from https://lifeinthefastlane.com (assessed May 29, 2018).

Burns, Edward. (2007). *Sinus rhythm with first degree block and PVC.* Retrieved from https://lifeinthefastlane.com (assessed May 29, 2018).

Burns, Edward. (2007). *Sinus rhythm with T-wave inversion.* Retrieved from https://lifeinthefastlane.com (assessed May 29, 2018).

Chapter 6

Burns, Edward. (2007). *Complete heart block.* Retrieved from https://lifeinthefastlane.com (assessed September 12, 2018).

Burns, Edward. (2007). *High lateral STEMI.* Retrieved from https://lifeinthefastlane.com (assessed September 7, 2018).

Chapter 6 *(Continued)*

Burns, Edward. (2007). *Inferior STEMI*. Retrieved from https://lifeinthefastlane.com (assessed September 7, 2018).

Burns, Edward. (2007). *Inferior STEMI with reciprocal change*. Retrieved from https://lifeinthefastlane.com (assessed September 7, 2018).

Burns, Edward. (2007). *Inferior STEMI with reciprocal change anterio-septally*. Retrieved from https://lifeinthefastlane.com (September 12, 2018).

Burns, Edward. (2007). *Left bundle branch block*. Retrieved from https://lifeinthefastlane.com (assessed September 12, 2018).

Burns, Edward. (2007). *LMCA infarction*. Retrieved from https://lifeinthefastlane.com (September 7, 2018).

Burns, Edward. (2007). *Posterior infarction*. Retrieved from https://lifeinthefastlane.com (assessed September 7, 2018).

Burns, Edward. (2007). *Proximal LAD occlusion*. Retrieved from https://lifeinthefastlane.com (assessed September 15, 2018).

Burns, Edward. (2007). *Right ventricular infarction*. Retrieved from https://lifeinthefastlane.com (assessed September 7, 2018).

Burns, Edward. (2007). *Septo-anterior NSTEMI*. Retrieved from https://lifeinthefastlane.com (assessed September 12, 2018).

12-LEAD EKG REFERENCE

Lead I **LATERAL** HIGH LEFT CIRCUMFLEX ARTERY	Lead aVR *SKIP INITIALLY* LEFT MAIN CORONARY ARTERY	Lead V₁ **SEPTAL** LEFT ANTERIOR DESCENDING ARTERY (SEPTAL BRANCH)	Lead V₄ **ANTERIOR** LEFT ANTERIOR DESCENDING ARTERY
Lead II **INFERIOR** RIGHT CORONARY ARTERY	Lead aVL **LATERAL** HIGH LEFT CIRCUMFLEX ARTERY	Lead V₂ **SEPTAL** LEFT ANTERIOR DESCENDING ARTERY (SEPTAL BRANCH)	Lead V₅ **LATERAL** LOWER LEFT CIRCUMFLEX ARTERY
Lead III **INFERIOR** RIGHT CORONARY ARTERY	Lead aVF **INFERIOR** RIGHT CORONARY ARTERY	Lead V₃ **ANTERIOR** LEFT ANTERIOR DESCENDING ARTERY	Lead V₆ **LATERAL** LOWER LEFT CIRCUMFLEX ARTERY

FRONTAL LEADS ⟷ HORIZONTAL LEADS

About the Author

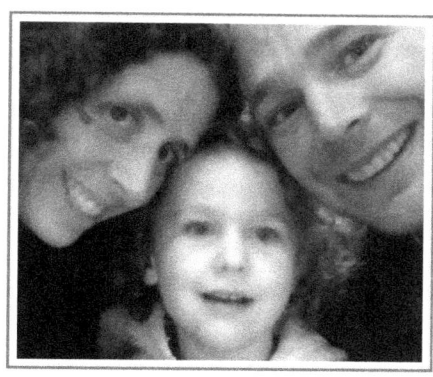

Nick Entsminger has been involved in the emergency medical services since 1997, working in frontier, rural, urban, and metropolitan venues for paid and volunteer 911 response. He's assisted in training paramedics, flight nurses, emergency medical technicians, and firefighters for more than 18 years as a lecturer, proctor, and field training officer. His advocation of EKG education stems from the lessons and knowledge he's gained through direct patient care and feedback from his peers. Mr. Entsminger believes in the shortcomings of ego and the power of knowledge advocating that skills can be learned from anyone, regardless of their education, trade, or title.

Nick currently lives in Northern California on a 22-acre homestead with his daughter and loving wife of more than 10 years. His hobbies include parenting, travel, carpentry, running, drumming, research, writing, teaching, and "B" action movies. He currently works as an EMS Specialist with a local EMS authority, assisting with policy development, trauma center designation, and other special projects.

www.ingramcontent.com/pod-product-compliance
Lightning Source LLC
Chambersburg PA
CBHW061756290426
44109CB00030B/2875